A COMPEND

OF THE

NEW MATERIA MEDICA

TOGETHER WITH

ADDITIONAL DESCRIPTIONS

OF SOME

OLD REMEDIES

BY

WM. H COOK, A. M., M. D.

CHICAGO:
PUBLISHED BY WM. H. COOK.

THE NEW MATERIA MEDICA.

THERAPEUTICAL CONSIDERATIONS.

Within the last few years the number of new agencies that have been brought before the medical profession is remarkable. On every side, and from every section of the globe, they have come in quantities, till the physician begins to feel embarrassed by the very richness of his medicamenta.

Experienced practitioners know that the most skillful physician usually employs but a limited number of remedies. Success in curing is gained by an intimate acquaintance with the exact powers of a few. and then the correct employment of these. Inexact knowledge of a multitude of articles and their employment in an uncertain and a haphazard manner bring little satitsfaction. Yet the physician needs to he informed of every means that properly can be made available in his calling. He wants to be familiar with whatever is reliable in his warfare against disease, and to have at his command the knowledge that will enable him to use any suitable measure. Not every article brought into notice has sustained the claims offered with it. No small number of them were found unworthy, and within a few months of their appearance were relegated to oblivion. Others arc undergoing scrutiny, and are but in the developmental stage. with nothing certain about them, and possibly on the way to early rejection. It is not desirable to burden a book with uncertain material, nor to pad out its bulk with magazine reports that have not yet been verified. In these busy days the physician wants that which has been tried and proven, leaving for his greater leisure and for the pages of the journals the further discussion of undetermined questions. Such a purpose has been kept steadily in view in this volume, both in presenting the new and in adding to the general stock of knowledge regarding the old.

The interests of science demand that all the evidence relating to a new article, that which militates against it as well as that which favors it, shall he recorded faithfully. Science is hindered, not promoted, by crowding upon the physicians attention a mass of ex parte and warmly-colored testimony in behalf of a new agent. Medical men weary of such testimony, and cautionsly await further information from which to form their judgment This is the conservative course of safety, by which the errors of a too-hasty acceptance are avoided and the advantages of a discriminating acceptance are gained.

In adjusting the balances of scientific discrimination, all agents may be classed as either Non-toxic or Toxic. This classification has been made in the present volume, and accords with the prevailing sentiment of the profession. One of the most common inquiries of physicians about a new article touches its toxicity, and upon the clinical answer given to that inquiry depends the future use of the agent. The earnestness of this questioning is understood by dealers, who commonly announces with each new article that it is non-toxic, or at least not so toxic as the one offered by another house, which it is expected to replace. Too often the outcome proves it to be highly toxic and unworthy of the confidence asked for it. The profession, ever humane, honorable and conscientious, resents thus being trilled with and made a party to incorrect announcements. Hence this firm separation of agents into toxic, and non-toxic classes is called for by the dictates of humanity and the interests of science.

Some prominence is here given to vegetable remedies native to our own country. This is believed to be the surest and most inviting road toward a higher and better Therapeutics. In the early part of this century such eminent scholars as Prof. Bigelow of Boston, Prof. Barton of Philadelphia, Prof. Ives of Yale, and other prominent medical gentlemen, took pride in seeking to develop our American Medical Botany. In this they sought to continue and to enlarge the labors of Rufinesque; and to follow the learned examples of Lindley, of Woodsville, of Stephenson and Churchill, and others in England.

So large anti rich are the resources of our American Medical Botany that the exploration of this vast Thesanrus has scarcely begun. While that which is good and worthy from other countries should be received gladly, that which is best and most worthy at our own door merits the first appreciative recognition. All this recognition is most deserved at the present time, when the products of foreign laboratories are pushed vigorously upon our attention, and the fabrications of chemical synthesis are candidate for the highest places. All due credit to pharmaceutical skill when it furnishes something really good.

But when so much that has come from the laboratory is worthless, and so much is toxic-and the highest claim of synthesis is a supposed imitation of what Nature has more perfectly prepared in some vegetable remedy-it is palpably to the advantage of the profession to turn aside from the crucibles of the laboratory and again look to the reliable products of Nature as did Bigelow, Barton and Ives.

In pharmacy the number of fluid extracts has increased to largely that nearly every vegetable agent is now offered in that form, and the dosee of a fluid extract is commonly taken as the standard for the agent. For purposes of dispensing this is a convenience, and is so generally accepted that crude or powdered drugs are not easily procured now. The advantages of prompt action from an infusion are thus often missed; for a fluid extract added to warm water is but a sorry imitation of an infusion; yet the neatness and uniform potency of the pharmaceutical preparation are more acceptable than the older mode of dispensing.

Fluid extracts have also largely supplanted the once popular powdered alcoholic extract called “Concentrated Remedies". For effectiveness in pill or capsule and convenience in making solutions many of these were admirable. Their too-common attenuation with starch or lactin brought their uniformity of strength under suspicion, and aided in effecting their retirement. Gain has been made, however, in the way of furnishing medicaments in smaller doses than pertained to the “heroic" past.; and parvules, granules and tablets have many advantages in the numerous cases where small doses at brief intervals accomplish more than large doses at longer intervals.

It is to be regretted, on the other hand, that manufacturing houses, while doing much that is praiseworthy, frequently issue preparations most unwisely put together. Agents of diverse actions are incorporated, desirable agents associated with thoroughly objectionable ones, and old-time standard preparations added to or rechristened in an unwarranted manner. So extensively are these methods followed in the greed for com-mercial gain that the pharmacist in his counting-house attempts to dictate the prescriptions of the physician a thousand miles from him. It is the fault of the profession if such assumptions are encouraged. A physician should scrutinize every compound offered to him, and reject everything not in accord with his own judgment, and refuse to deal out anything containing an agent he does not approve, and that might jeopardize a life for which he, and not the manufacturer, is responsible. No medical man should for a moment place his professional intelligence in the keeping of the druggist, but should discriminate rigidly in the preparations offered to him, and not allow himself or his patients to fall victims to unjustified and merely commercial combinations of drugs.

These considerations have been kept in view in preparing this volume. There is much unrest in the medical world at this time. It is felt that the entire science of Therapeutics is in process of revision; and that whatever is ungrounded is to be put aside, and a basis found that will endure without fluctuating. Fluctuation is an evidence of weakness; durability is secured only by carefully building upon facts that cannot be moved. This volume seeks to give accurate information, discriminating cautiously rather than reaching conclusions hastily.

PART I.

NON-TOXIC AGENTS

ACIDUM BORICUM

BORIC ACID-BORACIC ACID

This acid is obtained now from the Borax of California by decomposing its solution with hydrochloric Acid. It comes to the market in fine, white, soft, odorless and light plates, somewhat unctuous to the touch, of a feeble acid reaction. Dissolves in 25 parts cold water, 3 parts boiling water, and readily in alcohol, ether and volatile oils. Hot glycerine dissolves large quantities of it, and this becomes a crystalline mass when cold-*Boro-glyceride.*

Medical Properties.-Similar in action to borax, but more powerful. It is seldom given to the stomach, but is mostly employed in washes and for its antiseptic effects. A saturated solution has been used on foul ulcers, erysipelas, thrush, as a spray in diphtheria, etc., soon removing the odor and soothing burning sensations; also in foul leucorrhoera and cervical ulcerations. One to ten grains to the ounce of water is a favorite with many oculists in purulent and other ophthalmias, and in offensive discharges from the ear. Boro-glyceride solution is used to advantage on the mucous surfaces, and is soothing, cleansing and a good antiseptic. Its impalpable powder, one part first rubbed well with some ether, may be made into an ointment with two parts each of spermuceti and sweet oil and one part white wax, melted.

ACTEA SPICATA.

HERB CHRISTOPHER, BANEBERRY.

A low perennial shrub of the order Ranunculacea, common in Europe. For centuries the root and berries have been a remedy among the people of England. Bitter and rather acrid in taste, stimulant and harsh in action. Used in obstinate constipation, small doses procuring early and free stools; large doses causing some griping, nausea and thin evacuations. Its action is not unlike that of podophyllum, and I much doubt its desirability.

ADEPS LANAE.

LANOLIN, WOOL FAT.

Wool, as taken from the sheep, contains a large amount of fat, which has to he removed before the wool can be used. Formerly this was washed away; now it is separated by first dissolving out the fat with benzine, evaporating this, treating the product with a weak alkaline solution, and from this soapy compound obtaining the fat. The unpurified fat is called *Agnine.*

Wool fat is soft, ointment-like, nearly white; usually coming to market mixed with 30 percent of water, and of a pale straw or orange color. It has the peculiar property of being miscible with twice its weight of water without changing its character and the addition of one-tenth of one percent of borax to the slightly-warmed lanolin will enable it to absorb five or more parts of water. Its most valued property is that of being rapidly absorbed by the skin, leaving the surface firmer and nearly dry. This quality makes it of great service when it is desirable to feed a fatty substance to the system by way of the skin, as in neurasthenia, tuberculosis, tabetic emaciation, etc. It may be used alone for this purpose, or incorporated with from one to five times its own weight of cocoanut oil, which is thus rendered more absorbable. Incorporated with lard, it is less rapidly absorbed.

This property of wool fat is utilized in making various ointments for skin medication, the agents dissolved in it being the more readily carried into the tissues.

For such purposes, the usual hydrated lanolin of the market is preferable to the white article containing no water; and it is often an advantage to warm (not melt) the fat and rub into it 50 to 75 percent. more water. Of many preparations of this kind, the following may be named, the figures representing parts:

Cold Cream.-Borax 2, liquid neutral soap 1, lanolin 20, rosewater 180, tinct. benzoin 1.

Cooling Ointment.-Lanolin 20, rose water 30, zinc oxide 10.

For Chillblains-Camphor 3, balsam Peru 1, oil almonds 16, adeps lanae and rose water, each 20.

Eczema Paste, Soft.-Zinc oxide and French chalk, each 2, olive oil and lime water, each 6, lanolin 4, tinct. benzoin 1.

Eczema Paste, Hard.-Oxide zinc 6, sulphur 4, fullers earth 2, lanolin anti benzoin, each 14.

Boric Acid Ointment.-Boric Add 2, lard 5, lanolin 18.

For Urethritis.--Almond oil 10, lanolin 40, hydrastia sulphate 1 to 3, water 300 to 500. I offer this to the profession with great confidence.

In compounding these and similar preparations of lanolin, the following methods are necessary: :Mix oils and lanolin, and melt them slowly at a low heat; pour this mixture into a mortar heated moderately, and stir with a warm pestle; add this water at the same temperature, a little at a time, stirring constantly. When all have been thus incorporated, put the mortar where it will cool quickly, continue to stir, and when the mass has cooled to a soft paste pour at once into vials or boxes.

ALBOLENE.

Albolene is one of several liquid products of the petrolatum class of an oily and unctuous nature, white, odorless, bland, and more readily absorbed than vaseline or petrolatum. Like others of its class, it is softening and soothing to chapped and inflamed surfaces; and is an excellent base for ointments, not becoming rancid. It is used alone for spraying in nasopharyngeal diseases; or for dissolving eucalyptol, menthol, thymol and similar articles when these are required in diphtheria. scarlatina, and other nose and throat ulcerations. It is a desirable agent. Solid albolene resembles the white vaseline, and is used as a vehicle in preparing ointments.

ALOIN.

Almost from time immemorial aloes has been used in the practice of medicine; and its cathartic action on the rectutm and its stimulating influence on the uterus are well known. Its effective principle. aloin, has been used for a number of years, but formerly was of uncertain power. It is now, by better processes, obtained of uniform strength, and may he used instead of the resin, being also milder in action. Its small dose of one-fourth to one, half grain commends it for combination in pills.

ALPINIA GALANGA.

GALANGAL, TOOTHACHE WOOD.

From the East Indies come two varieties of galangal, one the Alpinia. and the other supposed to be the Maranta galanga; but it seems most probable that both are or the genus Alpinia. They come to market in cylindrical pieces three or four inches long, from the thickness of the little finger to that of the thumb, dull reddish-brown outwardly and orange-brown inwardly, fibrous. hard, of a pleasant aromatic odor and pungent taste.

Galangal is a stimulant, warming and aromatic, spicy and sharp, and rather permanent in its action. It has been much used like other aromatica stimulants, for toothache, and many people think highly of it for temporary relief. It is too exciting to the stomach for internal use except in conditions of decided local depression; but when such conditions exist, galangal will be found a prompt diffusive, and an infusion is useful in arousing circulation, promoting general and outward warmth, restoring suddenly-suppressed menstruation, breaking up colds, etc. It is usually best to employ it as a stimulating adjunct to less pungent articles, as asclepias, chamomile, ginger, and similar agents. In activity it resembles the bark of xanthoxylum, but is more agreeable to the taste.

ALSTONIA CONSTRICTA.

BITTER BARK, AUSTRALIAN FEVER BARK.

From Australia has come the bark of this shrub or small tree. of the apocynum family. It is yellowish brown, contains a dye, and is intensely bitter. Medicinally it is a stimulating tonic, influencing the general nerve structure, improving the secretions, and invigorating the circulation. It has been compared to cinchona, but lacks the astringent qualities of that agent. and more directly aids the digestive and secretory functions. It is suited to depressed and atonic conditions, and is a valuable agent of its class, So potent an article naturally has come to be used in intermittent typhoid and septic conditions, dropsy, and similar depressed circumstances. Dose, half a grain to two grains.

Alstonia Scholaris, called Dita Bark and Beng, is similar to A. Constricta. being a general tonic of the rather stimulating class. It is a reliable nerve tonic, and well calculated for use in malarial troubles. For a time it had a reputation in diarrhoea, dysentery, cholera, etc., but its uses in such maladies are secondary to its tonic influence.

AMPELOPSIS QUINQUEFOLIA.

AMERICAN IVY, VIRGINIA CREEPER.

This native climbing. woody plant is distinguished by its fine leaves radiating from a common centre. It grows wild over large sections of the country; and now is much cultivated for its hardy and rapid growth, covering fences and houses with beautiful green foliage from early spring, the leaves changing to brilliant crimson in the fall.

Medical Properties.-The bark and young twigs have acquired a good reputation as an alterative. They are largely re1axant and moderately stimulant, leaving behind a mild tonic impression, They act on the glandular system in general, including the lymphatics; and exert quite an influence on the salivary glands and mucous membranes, and some on the kidneys. By these qualities the drug has proven of service in scrofulous and syphilitic cases, especially as an associate of the more stimulating alteratives, as stillingia, A favorite compound is Rumex four parts, Celastrus two parts, Scrophularia and Ampelopsis each one part. It is a good adjunct to aralia hispida to increase the activity of the kidneys; and may be added to expectorants with advantage. Dose of the fluid extract, twenty drops to half a fluid drachm three or four times a day as an alterative.

AMPHIACHYRIS DRACUNULOIDES.

BROOM WEED.

From Texas has come this new remedial agent, as yet a little known member of the family Compositae. It seems to be abundant in some sections of the State and is described as a small, erect herb, 1 to a feet high, with numerous branches above and linear leaves with a strong midrib appearing almost like sessile bracts. Flowers small, yellow, in panicled racemes; rays 7 to 10, disk 13 to 18: blooms in autumn.

Medical Properties.-The leaves, flower heads and smaller branches are used medicinally; and earnest attention has been called to them by Dr. Massie, of Dallas. They appear to contain a gum-resinous material and a small amount of volatile oil; but no detailed examination of them has yet been made, beyond the fact that their gummy character makes it difficult to reduce them to powder, and a menstruum of 66 percent. alcohol is required to extract their qualities.

As a remedy, the article is an agreeable, a prompt and exceedingly diffusive stimulant, moderately sharp to the taste, influencing the mucous membrane of the larynx, trachea and bronchi quite decidedly, extending its impression to the stomach and intestines. It stimulates the capillary circulation, both inward and outward; thus relieving congestions of the mucous membranes, promoting warm perspiration, increasing expectoration, and sometimes leading to evacuations in acute intestinal catarrh. It also has a soothing and sustaining after-effect on the nerve peripheries, affording considerable relief from distresses of mucous surfaces by acting on the nerves as well as by relieving capillary distension and pressure.

Such properties make the agent a desirable one in many conditions where a pleasant and quickly diffusible stimulant is required. It holds a remedial position between ginger and xanthoxylum, without resembling either. Probably it will be found desirable as an adjunct to more positive and permanent agents, and its own effects are rather too transient to be effective in many cases. In flatulent colic, the tenesmus of diarrhoea and similar cases, it is an excellent antispasmodic and carminative. Its prompt action on the larynx makes it serviceable for relaxation of the vocal chords and the uvula, in aphonia from relaxation, and oedema glottidis.

In sub-acute and chronic bronchitis it procures a free dislodgment of vivid secretions, and relieves dyspnoea; and in offensive catarrhs is good, either as a snuff or a wash. It warms up the stomach, and will be a valuable adjunct to suitable agents in atonic dyspepsia. Its local use has been suggested in degenerate leucorrhea, and in many other connections where a moderate stimulant is required.

Combinations embracing this agent may he numerous, as is always the fact with a diffusive stimulant. Thus, to promote perspiration in colds, bronchitis, pneumonia, etc., it may be used with asclepias; in colic with dioscorea; in asthma, with lobelia for a cough and deficient expectoration, with aralia and palemonium. In these ways, the agent has a wide field of usefulness; and its good qualities make it worthy of considerable attention.

APIUM GRAVEOLENS.

CELERY.

Botanically Allied to parsley, the celery plant has long been esteemed for the edible character of its blanched and spiky leaves. These have a pleasant soothing effect on the nerves, and promote restfulness and sleep, diffusing a mildly sustaining impression through the system, Celery seeds, and in almost an equal measure the roots, have been introduced to medicine. Their action is that of an aromatic and quite diffusive nervine leaving a somewhat pungent taste and impress. They are used for the nervous system where a prompt soothing and mildly stimulating action is required. This makes them suitable in that large class of nervous cases where there is excitability with loss of tone, such as hysteria, insomnia, mild degrees of neurasthenia, etc. Their action is so diffusive that it is usually advisable to connect them with agents of a more permanent character, such as caulophyllum, scutellaria, dioscorea, and similar potent nervines. Celery often makes an agreeable and a desirable adjunct to such articles; but its influence is not sufficiently permanent to accomplish the desired object when given alone. The fluid extract of the seeds, in doses of from three to seven drops every three or four hours, represents them moderately well.

From being associated with other and apparently some dangerous. articles in sundry proprietary compounds, the celery is too often looked upon as fit only to be used in some secret nostrum.

APIUM PETROSELINUM.

PARSLEY.

Also called *Petroselinum sativum.* This common garden plant was introduced from Southern Europe, and is used for culinary purposes on account of the pleasant flavor of a small amount of volatile oil in its leaves. The entire plant contains some of this oil, about 4.25 percent. having been obtained by distillation from the seeds.

Apiol and *Apiolene* have been obtained recently from the seeds, and also from the roots. Apiolene is an oleo-resin, red or yellowish-red, resembling a fixed oil. but not modified by alkalies, wholly insoluble in water, soluble in alcohol and ether, of a pungent taste, having a peculiar and penetrating odor. It is obtained from the seeds by different processes, principally by first obtaining a saturated alcoholic tincture, concentrating this by evaporation, dissolving out the oleo-resin by ether, then filtering and evaporating. It is manufactured most extensively in France, and comes to the market in capsules containing about six drops.

Apiol is a colorless, crystalline substance, insoluble in water, soluble in alcohol, ether and the fixed oils; of a feeble parsley like odor. It comes on the market in fine needle-like crystals, or as white powder.

Medicinal Properties.-In my Dispensatory I spoke of parsley root as a diuretic, in which connection it deserves far more attention than it has received. Like many agents that act on the kidneys, it has been found to influence the nervous tissues und the female genitalia, and to be serviceable in relieving the reflex agitations of hysteria and in no small measure acting as an antispasmodic in certain cases of dysmenorrhea. A fluid extract of the seeds is prepared.

Apiolene represents chiefly the stimulating properties of the seed being only moderately relaxing. It influences the renal functions to but a small degree, and that secondarily through the nervous system. Its principal influence is upon the vaso-motor system of the reproductive organs, securing a more active circulation through the uterus and its appendages, at the same time relieving spasmodic tension to a moderate degree. It thus becomes serviceable in congestion and spasmodic dysmenorrhoea and secondarily in the general nervous disturbances connected with utero-ovarian congestion. By promoting the pelvic circulation it, becomes a stimulating emmenagogue, and is of use in deficient or delayed menstruation.

Not acting as a uterine tonic, its alleged power in atonic amenorrhoea will be found overrated; but it is, by its prompt action in filling and sustaining the uterine vessels, well adapted to many recent cases, and also in vicarious menstruation. It is said to stimulate the sexual powers somewhat.

Apiol represents the more relaxing powers of the seeds, and the stimulating in less degree. With this difference in properties, it is useful in dysmenorrhoea of the spasmodic class with decided advantage, and in hysteria; but is of less use in amenorrhoea. It, as well as apiolene, has been spoken of as an antiperiodic; but there is nothing of significance to bear out this claim. The fresh juice of parsley root, however, has some influence over the approaching paroxysms of an intermittent.

Apiol is given in doses of four grains twice or three times a day for dysmenorrhoea, beginning one or two days before the expected period. In very large doses it fills the cerebral vessels and causes temporary excitement and frontal headache. Apiolene in 6-drop capsules is used twice a day for amenorrhoea, beginning a week before the proper period, Both agents are of value in their respective places for diffusive action; but, as usual. the manufacturers overrate them.

APOCYNUM CANNABINUM.

WHITE INDIAN HEMP, NUNQUOT,

This member of the apocynum family is common near the banks of small streams from New England to Dacotah and south to Texas. It is much more abundant than its associate Apocynum androesemifolium or Black Indian Hemp; and though not the same in properties as the latter, is frequently given in its stead.

Medical Properties. I was familiar with this root in Central New York in 1853, Onondaga Indians using it as a remedy; and it was in use by the Cattamugus Indians in Western New York. My earlier employment of it found it to be a distinct stimulating tonic and diuretic, acting well upon the bowels, Further observation has confirmed this experience. Such properties make it of much service in renal and hepatic dropsies, as it fully opens the great emunctories of liver, bowels and kidneys, and gives them tone for the steady performance of their offices. It is an agent of potency, moderately prompt and quite persistent in action, and to be relied on. Dose of fluid extract as a laxative, 15 to 20 drops; as a diuretic, 3 to 5 drops every three hours.

Among other uses to which the New York Indians were said to put. it was in the bite of the rattlesnake, for which they consider it infallible. They scraped or bruised the fresh root and applied it to the wound; and then made an ounce of it into a pint of infusion, and gave two or three ounces of this every hour, and then every two hours.

ARBUTIN.

Arbutin is a glucoside principle found in both species of the uva ursi, and also in epigea repens, chimaphila, gaultheria. and some other plants. It comes to market as colorless. silken, needle-like crystals, soluble in 8 parts of cold water, less soluble in alcohol. Its action resembles that of uva ursi, but I have not found it so effective or reliable as the leaves. Its large dose of ten to fifteen grains does not make it an attractive remedy.

ARCTOSTAPHYLOS GLAUCA.

California furnishes this large evergreen shrub of the uva ursi family. The leaves are similar in properties to those of the old-time uva ursi, but are rather more pronounced in power. As an astringent of the tonic class they act well upon the mucous surfaces, strongly upon the bladder und urinary passages. They are much used in California for the laxity of diarrhoea; and have come into good professional repute for the later stages of gonorrhea and for gleet, and are used internally and as injection. In catarrh of the bladder and bloody urine they will be found reliable; and probably also in cbyluria, and for eneuresis, giving tone to the kidneys and the walls of the bladder. My observations suggest that the fluid extract does not represent the drug well, and that it is best used as infusion. The principle *arbutin* is found in these leaves.

ARECA CATECHU.

ARECA NUT, BETEL NUT.

An Asiatic palm of slender growth, this graceful tree is much cultivated for its beauty and for various purposes of utility to which its nut-like fruit is applied, as well as for its fragrant flowers.

Medically it is greatly valued by the natives; but seems to possess no higher properties than that of an astringent of the moderately tonic class. It is reputed a vermifuge for dogs: but it is doubtful if it exerts any vermifuge powers on man. Dose of fluid extract as a vermifuge, 2 drachms.

ARTEMISIA FRIGIDA.
MOUNTAIN SAGE. SAGE BUSH.

This is the little herb, a foot in height, that is so common on the eastern slope of the Rocky Mountains, and different varieties of which are distributed through Minnesota, Idaho. New Mexico and Texas. Though not botanically a1lied to the garden sage, it resembles it in flavor, and hence its popular name. In addition to its sage-like aroma, it has a rather lasting bitterness.

Medicinal Properties.-A warm infusion is stimulating and diffusive filling the superficial capillaries, increasing the action of the heart somewhat and promoting warm diaphoresia. Its influence on the vaso-motor system is quite decided, and has led to its use in malarial, typhoid and rheumatic fevers and scarlatina. A fair diuretic action is also obtained from it; and its use in congestive conditions in general is well attested. The fluid extract is used in amenorrhoea, pelvic engorgements with atony, rheumatism and diphtheria. Dose, half to a whole fluid drachm every three hours; given in hot lemonade when prompt action is desired.

ASPARAGUS OFFICINALIS.
ASPARAGUS.

The young shoots of this well-known garden plant, used as an edible, act promptly on the kidneys, soon effusing a disagreeable odor to the urine, sometimes excessively so when used freely: and leads to the elimination of an unusual amount of solids, my judgment being that the urates are mostly increased. It thus relieves the nervous system, heart and muscular tissues of the effects of retained renal elements; by which results it has been placed among the nervines and heart sedatives. It evidently has no direct action on the heart, but relieves by the valuable and natural process of eliminating toxic elements through the kidneys.

The promptness of its action makes it a useful associate with more stimulating and permanent diuretics, such as juniper and aralia hispida. A syrup is prepared from the fresh juice by heating, filtering. and then adding sugar. A fluid extract is on the market, of which the dose is twenty drops to half a fluid drachm three times a day. It is of use in renal dropsies: and I have found benefit from it in muscular forms of rheumatism.

Asparagin will be spoken of in the Appendix.

BALSAMODENDRON MYRRHA.
MYRRH.

From the earliest times, myrrh has been known in medicine as a stimulating emmonagogue and antiseptic. Its use has been restricted because its qualities make it unsuitable in sensitive and inflamed conditions of the stomach and bowels, and in all sthenic conditions. But in lax, atonic, degenerate, and gangrenous states, whether used outwardly or inwardly, it occupies It field of usefulness that it is safe to say no other remedy can fill. As an antiseptic, whether on the theory of destroying bacteria or simply as a preventive of decay, it is of unquestioned power. It was among the "spices" used in embalming the Pharaohs and nobles of Egypt, and was used alone to preserve indefinitely the bodies of the poor. An article that has prevented decomposition in the dead for 2,000 and 3,000 years is assuredly in the front rank among antiseptics.

Passing by the medical uses of myrrh which long have been known, I wish here to present some of my experiences with it in case where it has been too seldom employed. For local purposes it is effective and reliable wherever there are low grades of the destructive processes without adequate resistive circulation, and in septic tendencies and gangrenous or putrefactive threatenings. It changes the offensive discharges, increases the local urterial action, checks the progress of destruction and sets up a line of vital resistance. Inwardly it exerts a similar influence, and it will then he absorbed into the general circulation where, as Binz has shown, it rapidly increases the number of white blood-corpusles. thus fortifying the system against the encroachments of septic poisoning. These properties render gum myrrh a very desirable agent in atonie fermentative indigestion: certain classes of degenerate ulcers; in offensive discharges from the nostrils, throat, lungs, bowels, or uterus; and in such septic maladies as diphtherin, malignant scurlatina, puerperal septicemia, phlegmonous erysipelas, anthrax, etc.

On thoroughly indolent and on offensive ulcers, on anthrax and gangrenes. Powdered myrrh may be applied until local circulation has been obtained and the parts present a healthy action. Being an intense and a concentrated agent, but a moderate quantity is needed in many cases; and it is usually best to combine it with a large excess of hydrastis to sustain the local venous circulation. When the depression is unusually great, these may be aided by a tenth part or less of capsicum until arterial excitement has been aroused. Myrrh alone is sufficiently astringent to hinder the free escape of the discharges and this is obviated by its combination with Hydrastis and a little borax, both of which favor antisepsis. It is usually best to employ these as a paste, moistening the powders with water containing some glycerine. On syphilitic sores its action is not gratifying. It acts well upon eroding cervical ulcers with foul and ichorous discharges. On gangrenes, myrrh and capsicum may be applied *ad libitum.*

In offensive menstrum, leucorrheal and lochial discharges, it does good service; and may be applied in suppository or by tampon, being given internally every four or two hours as needed. Also given internally in puerperal septicaemia, phlegmons, threatening gangrene of the lungs and stomach. and similar dangers, accompanied by such sustaining articles as scutellaria and hydrastis in full quantities, In bronchiectasis and pulmonary cavities, advantage will be achieved from small doses several times a day.

For diphtheria, myrrh can be used locally and internally; and its antiseptic powers in this malady are most desirable, both upon the decaying exudate and when constitutional poisoning is imminent or has begun. Locally, one part of tincture with one part of glycerine and ten or more parts of water, makes an admirable spray when the exudate in the throat is gray or brown, the breath offensive and the nostrils are discharging foul material. Such a spray used thoroughly every two hours, with hydrogen peroxide between, is highly effective treatment Hydrastis and a small quantity of borax can be associated with the myrrh in such a spray to evident advantage. At the same time medium doses of myrrh should be given internally every three hours or oftener, associated with such other measures as are indicated, My favorite prescription is for a child of six years, two drops each tincture of myrrh and glycerine, one drop fluid extract hydrastis, in syrup every two hours. This liberal use of myrrh in this malady has proven remarkably successful in my practice for more than 25 years, giving results far more positive and uniform than any other treatment I have seen formulated. It is not a suitable agent to use in light cases with a bright color to the membranes, which are but on the borders of a simple ulceration; for these do not require the stimulating antiseptic measures that arc called for when the membranes are dusky and the exudate is prone to early decay.

Myrrh is too stimulating and drying to use as an antiseptic in typhoid; yet in a few cases with offensive stools, the tongue being moist, I have given it for a few days in one-grain doses every four hours with improvement of the discharges and a good subsequent history. In extreme typhoid tympanites, the bowels being closed by angulation, I have several times given two grains of myrrh with ten grains of fresh charcoal; and in a few hours realized the arrest of fermentation, reduction of tympanites and removal of occlusion, non-offensive passages occurring in from 6 to 10 hours.

In typho-malaria, small and very frequent vomiting may occur, black or greenish-black portions of pasty and offensive bile being ejected, and the stomach rejecting everything given. Considering the gastric, hepatic and other alvine secretions to be in a semi-putrescent state, this condition provoking the distressing vomiting, I have a number of times exhibited myrrh as an antiseptic. For this purpose, I rubbed together ten grains of myrrh in lump, twenty grains of lactin and five grains of soda bicarbonate, the latter aiding the solution of the myrrh. On this four ounces of hot water were poured, five drops of the fluid extract of cypripedium added as a nervine, and a teaspoonful given every 30 or 20 minutes. This would be retained, and soon check the vomiting; and in a few hours the mixture could be given at longer intervals. and the stomach would receive other remedies in divided doses. By the same method I have arrested other vomitings of septic origin.

The dose of from ten to thirty grains usually advised for myrrh, I believe to be entirely too large. Only in a few exceptional cases have I given so much as five grains as a dose; and have been most satisfied with the agent in doses of one to two grains, and half a grain at intervals of two hours or less is often best. The article is very concentrated in its powers and long-continued in its action, hence the advisability of small doses. Unlike most gum-resinous substances, its tincture added to water separates into milkiness without settling, which is an advantage in using it as a spray or in minute doses. The lump retains the volatile oil that is commonly lost in the powder.

BAPTISIA TINCTORIA.
WILD INDIGO.

Nearly thirty years ago I fully described this American plant as a peculiarly antiseptic and stimulating agent; and one that was an excellent application to degenerate ulcers, and a potent remedy in depressed conditions of the glandular system. It has been introduced recently as a "new" remedy, so prone is the profession to re-discover and laud what in the past they ignored or ridiculed.

Baptisia has fully sustained itself in the position I formerly gave it. As an antiseptic its influence is distinct, not wholly from a germicidal arrest of putrefaction, but mostly from its power of sustaining the local arterial circulation, and thus combatting the tendency to decay and preventing the absorption of decaying products. This makes it useful in foul ulcers of all kinds, offensive erysipelatous sores threatelling gangrene, diphtheritic sloughing, fetid leucorrhea and other discharges.

For local treatment in all such cases, it is strong and effective; and may be added in moderate proportions to hydrastis, prunus, and similar articles, or used in combination with borax, eucalyptus and other antiseptics. In degenerate scrofula and syphilis, it is a desirable addendum to arctium, sarsaparilla, and other rcelaxing alteratives. It is misplacing it to use it for antiseptic purposes in typhoid, for its local stimulation is too active. The agent is very potent, and a small portion answers the purpose loca1ly. Dose inwardly, 1 to 2 drops of fluid extract..

BENWINOL.

A heavy, colorless, oily liquid obtained from Pennsylvania petroleum without, as is claimed, the use of sulphuric acid or other chemical. A minute portion of benzoin is added, giving it a faint benzoic flavor; otherwise it is tasteless and odorless, without a trace of kerosene. It is liquid and unchangeable. Benzoinol is used for diseases of mucous surfaces, as of the nose, pharynx, bronchi, vagina and urethra. It is bland and soothing, spreading readily upon such surfaces and protecting them. Generally administered in spray, an atomizer reducing it to a very fine spray that easily reaches the tiny channels of the nasal and bronchial passages. Employed in catarrh, ozoena, pharyngitis, laryngitis, and ulcerations of these parts. Some use it in chronic bronchitis and bronchial asthma and to allay certain tickling coughs. Like some others of the petroleum class, it is suggested for internal as well as local use in early phthisis. Applied to the vagina on tampons, it allays inflammation and lessens the discharges of acute and sub-acute leucorrhoea. It has given favorable results as an injection in urethritis, cystitis, gonorrhoea, etc., where it cleanses the surfaces of tenacious discharges and leaves a soothing impression.

Benzoinol is a solvet for a number of articles useful in throat and nasal medication, such as eucalyptol, menthol, thymol, oils of pinus, tar, gaultheria and cubebs. Five to ten drops may be added to the ounce of benzoinol; and used as a spray or for purposes of inhalation. With hydrastia sulphate (grs. ij to ℥ j) it is useful in eczema, psoriasis and other inflammatory skin diseases.

BERBERIS AQUIFOLIUM.
OREGON GRAPE ROOT, HOLLY-I.EAVED BARBERRY, MOUNTAIN GRAPE.

From the Pacific slope has come this new remedy, the root being one of the most valuable additions to the rnedicamenta. Especial credit is due to Dr. J. H. Bundy, California, for bringing it before the profession; and to the house of Parke, Davis & Co. for their energy in obtaining and presenting it.

The article is an alterative of the tonic class, bitter and fairly stimulating, acting slowly and permanently. It extends its action throughout the glandular system and the lymphatics, gradually and steadily bringing about increased action and tone in all these structures. It thus improves appetite and digestion, promotes a better secretion and excretion of bile, sustains the secreting power of the kidneys and skin, and thus eliminates morbific retentions from the system. Such qualities place it among the potent articles of the materia medica, and make it serviceable in a large variety of cases.

Its most admirable use is in secondary and tertiary syphilis, and in the various ulcerations and scaly skin diseases of syphilitic origin. A professional acquaintance aptly calls it a "syphilis chaser"; and the results of its administration in all that class of maladies are very satisfactory. Similarly it is effective in scrofulous ulcer boils, and other troubles where glandular inaction has depraved the system.

It has been spoken of highly in non-inflammatory eczema, psoriasis, pityriasis and in all cutaneous affections and discolorations connected with hepatic derangements. Upon the portal system its action is quite direct, sustaining the portal circulation, and relieving the long train of symptoms following in the wake of torpid liver, jaundice and cholaemic poisoning. In the connection it improves certain forms of indigestion, relieves biliousness, and bilious headache, takes from the kidneys the burden of their attempt to eliminate the bile, and improves the action of the bowels without itself being a cathartic. For these purposes it is well used in combination with euonymus or cascara: while for the more general alterative purposes it is an excellent addition to preparations of ampelopsis, trifolium, sarsaparilla., etc. From its sustaining action on the liver, it is well adapted to chronic torpor, chronic hepatitis, malarial troubles, including "mountain fever," ague cake, etc. Dose of the fluid extract, 5 to 20 drops three or four times a day. The plant contains berberina and an alkaloid principle, but these have not been put on the market.

BIGNONIA CAROBA.

CAROBA.

The *Jacaranda Caroba* of DeCandolle, a goodly tree, native to Brazil, of the same family as our shrubby climbing Trumpet-flower, and the luxuriant Catalpa. It grows to a height of 30 or more feet, bearing dark-green compound leaves, each of the 10 or 12 elliptic leaflets being nearly 2 inches in length; flowers red and white, in large clusters, fragrant. The leaves are medicinal, and abound in various resins, some of which are agreeably balsamic, all soluble in alcohol. A fluid extract prepared from these leaves represents the combined virtues of their several resins and balsams; and its desirable qualities should be understood more fully by the profession. It is seldom known by any other than its Spanish name, Caroba.

Medical Properties.-A distinct balsamic stimulant with fair relaxing qualities, leaving a desirbhle astringing-tonic impression. It acts upon the entire excretory glandular system-skin, mucous surfaces, kidneys, and liver. This action is rather prompt, but also steady and prolonged. It thus proves to be a general depurator, agreeably promoting the elimination of poisonous and offensive materials, and leaving the system well invigorated. By virtue of these properties, it is an admirable agent in the treatment of venereal diseases-not from any mythical power to neutralize or antagonize the venereal virus, but from its ability to promote the successful elimination of the toxic matter through the normal functions. This is the one and only true way of curing syphilitic diseases and abundant experience proves that caroba leaves are among the best and most reliable agents for this purpose. It is pleasant to take, is withal a good stomachic tonic, and a truly valuable constitutional remedy.

In syphilitic and other skin diseases of the non-inflammatory class, it is excellent; and as a depurator by the skin and kidneys will be found of service in chronic rheumatism, and in scrofulous affection. Local applications are effective in stimulating all classes of foul, indolent and degenerate ulcers. For these purposes the fluid extract will be applied in severe cases: or made into an ointment with vaseline, 1 to 3 drachms to the ounce, for milder purposes. Dose of the fluid extract, 20 to 40 drops four times a day.

BISMUTH SUBGALLATE.

DERMATOL.

Subnitrate of bismuth has long been in use as an astringent and soothing article for irritable diarrhoea, sub-acute gastritis, pyrosis, gastric ulcer, and as a local application in irritable leucorrhoea and ulcers. Opinions differ as to its toxicity. some pronouncing it entirely harmless; but my own use of it has been too limited to decide the questions but the general literature of bismuth does not incline me in its favor.

Subgallate of bismuth, first offered under the name of Dermatol, is of recent introduction. It is a pale yellow powder, soft, inodorous, tasteless; insoluble in the usual menstrua. It is not so soothing as the subnitrate, but more antiseptie: and it seems quite favorably to arrest digestive fermentation and irritability in the bowels, and to correct unhealthy conditions in ulcers when dusted on them. Applied as a powder to surgical wounds or to other solutions of continuity, it is an un-irritating protective and antiseptic. It is thus free from both the irritating properties and the disagreeable odor which render some of the other antiseptics objectionable. It is, however, as a remedy in fermentative dyspepsia, and in affections accompanied by fermentation in the intestines that the salt has been most mentioned of late.

Dr. Austin Flint regards it as par excellence the remedy as functional disturbances referable to the stomach and bowels, and accompanied by flatulence and distress-more efficient than salicin and the salicylic acid salts, and free from the objections to the latter. He was led to its use by seeing it recommended as a valuable remedy in the diarrhorea of children, tiding as a disinfectant. He reports a number of cases in which the results following its use certainly bespeak it a valuable remedy in the class of cases indicated. Dose for an adult, 2 to 5 grains an hour after meals.

BORAGO OFFICINALIS.
BORAGE.

In Europe, where this plant is native, it was formerly held in much esteem; but the passion for more powerful agents gradually pushed it aside till it became almost unknown to the profession outside of France. Of late its use has been revived in America.

It is an annual, now cultivated for its fine blue flowers. All parts of the plant abound in mucilage, connected with mild and diffusive properties of the rather relaxing grade. An infusion is quite soothing to the bronchial surfaces and slightly diaphoretic; hence is useful in colds, recent coughs with bronchial irritation, measles, and similar conditions.

Like other relaxants and demulcents, it acts fairly on the kidneys and bladder, and thus increases urination and relieves cystitis, and is of service in recent cystic and vaginal catarrhs. A t one time it enjoyed a reputation in rheumatism, probably because of its diaphoretic and diuretic action. The infusion may be used freely; the fluid extract is given in doses of 10 to 30 drops three or four times a day.

CALENDULA OFFICINALIS.
MARIGOLD.

Garden marigold is well known to everybody. A century and more ago its flowers were a popular medicine, but fell into disuse as more powerful agents became fashionable; now their use is revived, and worthily so.

Marigold is mild in power, acting as a moderate stimulant and tonic on the nerves and capillaries. These properties make it an antispasmodic and, in warm infusion, a gentle diaphoretic. Indirectly it is useful in dysmenorrhrea and menstrual suppressions from cold. Its best use, however, is as a local application in bruises, sore muscles, sprains, and similar conditions; for which purpose the tincture is employed, and if preferable to arnica. It is also an excellent application in the ear for congestion, softness, discharges and similar relaxed conditions of the tympanum and other membranes. Used as a wash on varicose veins it strengthens them and reduces their size, and promotes the healing of varicose ulcers; and may be used internally at the same time. These results suggest that the article is a mildly astringent tonic to venous walls; and it may be found useful in passive uterine hemorrhages.

CAPSELLA BURSA-PASTORIS.
SHEPHERD'S PURSE, MOTHER'S HEART.

A very common plant, resembling the lepidium or pepper grass; but lacking the pungent taste of the latter, and having a layer of leaves close to the ground.

Medical Properties.-An old-time family medicine of pioneer days, and a favorite among some of the earlier botanic physicians, this insignificant weed has lately engaged considerable professional attention. It is a gentle stimulant, with mild tonic and astringent qualities, influencing the kidneys and bladder principally, also acting on the mucous membranes of the uterus and vagina. Its chief use is in catarrh of the bladder, congestion of the kidneys, sandy deposits in the urine, eneuresis, and similar renal troubles. For all such purposes it is an admirable remedy, and may be associated with agrimony, stigmata maidis, and similar articles. It is of service in gonorrhrea and gleet, and in various female weaknesses is a desirable associate for mitchella, viburnum, etc. It is somewhat of a stimulating expectorant. An infusion best represents the plant, and may be taken freely. Dose of fluid extract, 10 to 40 drops four or more times a day.

CARICA PAPAYA.
MELON TREE, PAPAW.

Our Northern papaw (Asimina triloba) is an entirely different tree from the Carica papaya, or papaw of the tropics. Carica is native to the West Indies and South America; but was carried to the East Indies, and now abounds there. It is a tree of about 20 feet, rising straight, with a round stem, crowned with leaves. The fruit is similar to a small melon; and as an article of food ranks almost equal to the banana, A milky juice abounds in the fruit, and in the trunk and leaves in smaller quantities. It is acid.

The unripe juice will soon ferment with butyric acid fermentation. On standing, a watery portion soon separates from a coagulated pulpy portion. From the watery portion may be precipitated, by alcohol, a white albuminous substance. The watery portion may be preserved by glycerine. The precipitate is now offered under the various names of papain, papoid, papayotin, and plant or vegetable pepsin. Of course it is carefully to be distinguished from the narcotic proprietary medicine papain.

Medical Properties. -When carica juice is unripe, it is a sharp irritant to the alimentary tract, causing drastic stools and often leading to inflammation. Papoid, as obtained from this juice, is an active digestant, much more potent and effective than pepsin. It acts vigorously on all classes of foods, best in the alkaline solution of the intestines, but with nearly equal thoroughness in the acid juices of the stomach; in which fact of not being influenced by either alimentary secretion it has a decided advantage over pepsin, which acts only in acid fluids. Papoid stimulates both the gastric and intestinal secretions. It dissolves mucous accumulations, promptly removing them in cases of gastric catarrh and of worms. It emulsifies fats, and converts starch into a form of maltose.

Its most suitable use is in atonic dyspepsia with deficiency of gastric juice, gastric catarrh with tenacious mucous accumulations, and intestinal indigestion with flatulence. It is not suitable in gastric or other irritation. Use has been made of it, locally, to dissolve the membrane of diphtheria, on indolent and foul ulcers where a half dead structure needs to be removed, etc. Some have suggested that it may attack the stomach itself, but there seems to be no good reason to think it will act on healthy living tissues. Dose 1 to 2 grains; the smaller dose being preferable. It may be given in tablet, or combined with pancreatin and soda bicarb.

CARUM COPTICUM.

AJOWAN, AJAVA SEEDS, LOVAGE.

In the East Indies the seeds of this umbelliferous plant have for many centuries been used as a condiment, and for a long time have had a place in their materia medica. It is a diffusive stimulant and carminative, leaving behind a slightly bitter and tonic impression. It is much stronger and more tonic than our caraway, to which it is allied. About 4 percent. of a volatile oil has been obtained from it, and this has yielded the antiseptic thymol. It is a desirable adjuvant in many conditions; and has an empirical repute in cholera and for dipsomania.

CAULOPHYLLUM THALICTROIDES.

BLUE COHOSH, PAPPOOSE ROOT.

Also classed as Leontice thalictroides. This native remedy has been much neglected by the profession, being too flippantly passed by as a nearly useless article; whereas it is a strong and valuable agent, and deserving of especial attention. The root is a nervine of the stimulating class, with moderate relaxing properties and a small amount of mucilage, somewhat prompt and decidedly positive in action. Such qualities, expended chiefly upon the nervous structures, make this cohosh a fine sustaining article in conditions of weariness and depression, and for neurasthenia in general. A large portion of its influence is directed toward the uterus, making it a most serviceable remedy in dysmenorrhcea and menstrual deficiency or suppression. It gives tone to the uterus and invigorates its circulation, while sustaining its nerve force and acting as an antispasmodic. In the various female troubles where an influence of this peculiar kind is needed, caulophyllum is a thoroughly reliable agent. It is commonly associated with viburnum and Mitchella.

Its common name of pappoose root suggests the use made of it by the aborigines. To sustain the uterine contractions in labor, and to give them regularity and steadiness, I believe there is nothing equal to it among the many agencies that have abounds in the fruit, and in the trunk and leaves in smaller quantities. It is acid.

The unripe juice will soon ferment with butyric acid fermentation. On standing, a watery portion soon separates from a coagulated pulpy portion. From the watery portion may be precipitated, by alcohol, a white albuminous substance. The watery portion may be preserved by glycerine.

The precipitate is now offered under the various names of papain, papoid, papayotin, and plant or vegetable pepsin. Of course it is carefully to be distinguished from the narcotic proprietary medicine papame.

Medical Properties. -When carica juice is unripe, it is a sharp irritant to the alimentary tract, causing drastic stools and often leading to inflammation. Papoid, as obtained from this juice, is an active digestant, much more potent and effective than pepsin. It acts vigorously on all classes of foods, best in the alkaline solution of the intestines, but with nearly equal thoroughness in the acid juices of the stomach; in which fact of not being influenced by either alimentary secretion it has a decided advantage over pepsin, which acts only in acid fluids. Papoid stimulates both the gastric and intestinal secretions. It dissolves mucous accumulations, promptly removing them in cases of gastric catarrh and of worms. It emulsifies fats, and converts starch into a form of maltose. Its most suitable use is in atonic dyspepsia with deficiency of gastric juice, gastric catarrh with tenacious mucous accumulations, and intestinal indigestion with flatulence. It is not suitable in gastric or other irritation. Use has been made of it, locally, to dissolve the membrane of diphtheria, on indolent and foul ulcers where a half dead structure needs to be removed, etc. Some have suggested that it may attack the stomach itself, but there seems to be no good reason to think it will act on healthy living tissues. Dose 1 to 2 grains; the smaller dose being preferable. It may be given in tablet, or combined with pancreatin and soda bicarb.

CARUM COPTICUM.

AJOWAN, AJAVA SEEDS, LOVAGE.

In the East Indies the seeds of this umbelliferous plant have for many centuries been used as a condiment, and for a long time have had a place in their materia medica.
It is a diffusive stimulant and carminative, leaving behind a slightly bitter and tonic impression. It is much stronger and more tonic than our caraway, to which it is allied. About 4 percent of a volatile oil has been obtained from it, and this has yielded the antiseptic thymol. It is a desirable adjuvant in many conditions; and has an empirical repute in cholera and for dipsomania.

CAULOPHYLLUM THALICTROIDES.

BLUE COHOSH, PAPPOOSE ROOT.

Also classed as Leontice thalictroides. This native remedy has been much neglected by the profession, being too flippantly passed by as a nearly useless article; whereas it is a strong and valuable agent, and deserving of especial attention. The root is a nervine of the stimulating class, with moderate relaxing properties and a small amount of mucilage, somewhat prompt and decidedly positive in action. Such qualities, expended chiefly upon the nervous structures, make this cohosh a fine sustaining article in conditions of weariness and depression, and for neurasthenia in general. A large portion of its influence is directed toward the uterus, making it a most serviceable remedy in dysmenorrhoea and menstrual deficiency or suppression. It gives tone to the uterus and invigorates its circulation, while sustaining its nerve force and acting as an antispasmodic. In the various female troubles where an influence of this peculiar kind is needed, caulophyllum is a thoroughly reliable agent. It is commonly associated with viburnum and Mitchella.

Its common name of pappoose root suggests the use made of it by the aborigines. To sustain the uterine contractions in labor, and to give them regularity and steadiness, I believe there is nothing equal to it among the many agencies that have been offered for this purpose. It has all the good qualities ever claimed for ergot; and not one of the latter's objectionable and dangerous qualities to either the mother or the child. Having used it largely in this connection for forty years, I am justified for speaking in warmest terms of its value as an aid in parturition. I have never known it to fail in any case; and have with it succeeded in arousing full uterine contractions and promoting early delivery, when the uterine inertia seemed hopeless. By preference, I use it as an infusion for these purposes; and if one-half part of myrica cerifera bark is associated with it, the effect will be all the more speedy and positive; and so true will be the uterine contractions that post-partum hemorrhage will very seldom occur, and will be controlled promptly by these agents. Physicians who will acquaint themselves with this use of caulophyllum, will soon find it a most potent remedy. When the pulse is small or is otherwise feeble, capsicum should be associated with it liberally, pro re nata, till full cardiac action has been secured.

As an antispasmodic, caulophyllum is of much service in puerperal convulsions and merits careful study in that connection. It may then be given in very large doses by enema, especially in company with lobelia; the enemas being introduced above the strait when possible, so as to be retained and effect their purpose. Small portions added to aralia, prunus and similar pectorals. are desirable in old and spasmodic coughs and bronchial irritations.

Dose of fluid extract, 2 to 5 drops every two hours in most cases; half a fluid drachm every hour or oftener in parturition.

CEREUS GRANDIFLORUS.

NIGHT-BLOOMING CEREUS, TORCH THISTLE.

Cereus Bonplandii of many botanists. Cactus grandiflorus of Linne. One of the lovely cacti indigenous to Mexico and southward. Several species of the same genus seem to possess identical properties.

Medical Properties.- Within a few years the stems of this plant have been introduced to therapeutics as a remedy for functional palpitation and other irregularities of the heart. Opinions were somewhat conflicting, probably from a misapprehension of the especial action of the article. If used in the hope of influencing the heart muscle, there will not be disappointment; and for purposes of sustaining the heart nerves and the respiratory nerves, it is effective and reliable. Such cardiac disturbances frequently result, indirectly, from sundry indigestions, uterine and ovarian affections, anaemia and other maladies and influences that exhaust the heart power and produce in this organ an irregular, intermitting or other improper, weak or tumultuous action. And accompanying the heart disturbance, as secondary to it, will be more or less dyspnoea, feelings of distress about the heart itself, dizziness, headache, impaired vision of amaurotic character, etc.

In all these instances, this cactus has been found an admirable agent and of prompt action. It directly sustains the nerves of the vaso-motor system, with a preference to those of the heart itself; and extends through the sympathetic system.

It thus becomes a tonic to the entire circulatory apparatus when this and its centre show evidences of failing strength, and becomes an invaluable adjunct in the treatment of many chronic and acute maladies, while due attention is being given to any primary and provocative disorder of the stomach, uterus, bowels, or other parts. It is also of value in neuralgias, not from supposed "sedative" properties, but because it invigorates the nerves, which are so generally depressed in neuralgias. By virtue of this power it increases general nerve tone, and has been used in tic doloreaux, angina pectoris, etc. So far as a "sedative" influence is desired in neuralgia, its use would be a failure; but on the principle of sustaining suffering nerves when depressed or exhausted, it will be found excellent. Its action is prompt, but rather transient. Keep this cactus to its true place, and it is most admirable. The fluid extract, in doses of 10 to 30 drops three times a day, or 5 drops at shortened intervals, pro re nata, is the most reliable form. A so-called active principle, cactina, is made into pellets; dose one to three every three or two hours.

In this connection mention may be made of the cereus tuberosa, a tuberous-rooted cactus of Mexico. The tubers, tinctured in diluted alcohol, are prized by the natives in the treatment of rheumatism, being applied locally with friction and taken internally. It is very indefinite to speak of an article as being good for rheumatism, unless some information is given as to its manner of securing benefit in that malady; yet this cactus deserves attention, for some particular merit generally underlies a strong popular belief in an article.

CHELIDONEUM MAJUS.

CELANDINE.

Both the herb and roots of celandine have been used in medicine, more by the people than by physicians. From the stem is obtained a juice that, when fresh, is an acrid stimulant; and has been used to remove corns and warts by stimulating them to exfoliation; and to destroy the parasite of itch. The dried herb and roots are stimulant, exciting the glands in general, sometimes sharply cathartic, moderately diuretic and expectorant. They have a decided action on the gall ducts and cyst, making them serviceable in depressed and catarrhal forms of jaundice. Some have valued the article in scrofulous affections, others to stimulate expectoration in old coughs, and yet others have used the juice in the eyes to remove pterygion.

Poisonous properties have been attributed to it, but it seems this is questionable; yet it is a harsh article, and needs further investigation before condemning or fully accepting it. Of the root, three ounces tinctured on a pint of diluted alcohol may be given in doses of a teaspoonful three times a day.

CISSAMPELOS PAREIRA.

PAREIRA BRAVA.

Chondodendron tomentosum, Cocculus chondodendron. It seems that three separate genera in the menispermum family furnish the root known in the market as pareira. The article comes from the warm latitudes, mostly from Brazil. It contains some resin; and a bitter principle called cissampeline or perosine, which is insoluble in water but soluble in alcohol, ether and acids.

Medical Propepties.-Pareira has enjoyed considerable repute as a tonic diuretic with aperient properties. It is somewhat stimulant, and decidedly bitter. Its action is chiefly on the renal organs, relieving congestion, increasing the amount of urine moderately, and acting very beneficially in chronic cystic catarrh. It also acts moderately on the gall cyst and ducts, excreting bile and leaving a tonic impression. These qualities have led to its use in dropsy, jaundice, and indirectly for rheumatism. Dose of the fluid extract, 20 to 40 drops three times a day.

CYPERUS ARTICULATUS.

ANTI-EMETW ROOT, ADRUK

Adrue belongs to the family of Rushes, this particular species abounding in the tropics. In the West Indies it is a remedy of the people for the arresting of vomiting in yellow fever, a decoction of the knobbed root being given in small and frequent doses. Its popularity attracted professional attention, and many excellent reports in its favor have been made. It is an aromatic of agreeable flavor, somewhat stimulating in action, warming to the stomach. It is reputed to be so effective in arresting vomiting, that even the vomiting of pregnancy promptly yields to it. That, with its use by some physicians for whooping cough, suggests that it combines relaxing with its stimulating properties, thus placing it among the antispasmodics.

It will be found a good stimulating nervine addendum to tonics in atonic dyspepsia, and to uterine tonics in menstrual derangements. The dose of the fluid extract is 5 to 20 drops every four hours or oftener.

DIPTEROCARPUS TURBIN ATUS.

GURJUN.

Bengal and other sections of India abound in several species of Dipterocarpus, all of which are immense and beautiful trees. From incisions in the bark there exudes an oleo-resin, of which fully 60 percent can be distilled over. This oleo-resin is known as gurjun balsam, gurjun oil and wood oil. It is a thick, brownish-yellow copaiba-like fluid, of not unpleasant resinous odor, and less objectionable to the stomach than the latter article. It is a stimulant and moderate astringent to the genito-urinary passages: used in blenorrhagia, gonorrhrea, chronic vaginitis, and similar cases, as copaiba is used. It is usually given in emulsion, or in capsules, 10 drops being a full dose. One part of gurjun balsam and two parts of lime water have been used on prepared cotton as a local application for subacute and chronic vaginitis; and some report the successful use in leprosy of a similar preparation, applied to the surface twice a day.

ECHINACEA PURPUREA.

PURPLE CONEFLOWER, BLACK SAMPSON.

A member of the Composite family, formerly placed in the genus Rudbeckia, closely allied botanically to the small wild sunflower and Black-eyed Susan of the Western States. Echinacea is common from Illinois and Wisconsin southward to Texas, on open prairies with a sandy soil, and around marshy spots. It is a slender plant from 2 to 3 feet high, rarely branched, stems mostly smooth, long, narrow and rough leaves, mostly on the lower part of the stem, thus placing the flower heads on long and naked peduncles. The centre or disk of the flower head rise,; cone-like, studded with small purplish flowers, and bearing a stiff chaff. Ray florets 15 to 20, one to two inches long, dull purple rarely inclining to whitish, turning downward so as almost to circle toward the stem. The top dies down each fall, but the root is perennia1. Root thick, black. Flowers in July and August.

Medical Properties.-Under its common name of Black Sampson, the roots of this Echinacea, and also of the E. Angustifolia, have enjoyed much popular repute as a medicine. They are quite pungent to the taste, not unlike the bark of Xanthoxylum, and leave a warm and somewhat bitter impression. They are among the rather decided stimulants, moderately diffusive, exciting the outward circulation, increasing the flow of saliva largely, and more gradually reaching the general glandular system. A warm infusion promotes diaphoretics rather freely, which has led to its popular use in snake bites. As an adjunct to the usual alteratives it will be found a valuable stimulant to the secernants in degenerate scrofulous conditions, scrofulous and similar chronic ulcers, fever sores, and secondary syphilis, in all which connections it can be relied on to promote the function of elimination throughout the system and to sustain the circulation in the arterioles. I offer the following formula as trustworthy in secondary syphilis and strumous cachexy:

Compound Syrup Echinacea. Roots of echinacea, lappa major and smilax pseudo-china, each four ounces; celastrus scandens and juniper berries, each two ounces. A half gallon syrup may be made of these in the usual way; dose, a drachm three or four times a day.

In diphtheria this agent has been used as an alleged antiseptic; but it arrests decay of membrane only as it sustains local circulation, and for this purpose it is useful. It may be used as a wash or ointment in all degenerate sores. Dose of the fluid extract, 5 to 20 drops.

ELECTRICITY.

Electricity as a physical agent may be advantageously employed in the treatment of certain forms of disease. Its proper use, and the methods of its application, depend upon a knowledge of its peculiarities and of the character of its actions in the human system under various circumstances. Many theories have been advanced regarding the exact nature of electricity; but it can be described only by its effects, and in terms which are convenient although merely figurative.

Its chief effect is the creation of molecular disturbance in and about bodies upon which it acts; the extent and character of the disturbance depending upon the degree and manner of application. Electrical manifestations may he produced by various means, such as heat, friction and chemical action. For medical purposes, electricity is usually generated by employing a "battery cell." The simplest form of cell is a glass jar containing dilute sulphuric acid in which a plate of zinc and a plate of copper are partially submerged.

The zinc is the more vigorously attacked by the acid; and by connecting the plates by a wire outside the jar, the molecular disturbance (called electricity) passes through the liquid from zinc to copper, and then along the wire from copper to zinc, forming what is termed a "voltaic circuit." Should a wire lead from the copper plate to a body, such as the human body, am} another wire from that body to the zinc, the molecular disturbance will be transmitted through the body from the copper plate to the wire leading to the zinc plate. This is the principle of the use of electricity in medicine.

The movement of electricity along the wire leading from the copper plate to the body is known as the positive or plus current; and that along the wire from the body to the zinc plate as the negative or minus current. The direction of the current is from the positive to the negative. The cell is termed a voltaic couple, or clement; and a battery composed of one or more such cells is called a galvanic battery when the current is employed directly. Accumulations of gas upon the copper, or impurities of the zinc (causing local currents-" polarization"), may temporarily destroy the effectiveness of a battery. The gas is easily removed by exposure, and the zinc may be rendered as though pure by covering (amalgamating) it with quick silver. Frequently some other element is substituted for copper, and contrivances have been invented as "constant" batteries to avoid temporary arrest of the current.

Daniell's, Grove's, and Bunsen's constant batteries are typical of those employing two elements and two liquids. The Leclanche cell consists of a carbon rod in a porous pot packed with manganese peroxide and gas graphite, and covered with pitch, the carbon being attached to a piece of lead to which the positive wire is fastened; the pot is set in a jar containing a solution of salammoniae in which is a zinc rod connected with the negative wire.

Kidder's battery cell consists of zinc and platinum plates in diluted sulphuric acid. The zinc-carbon-bichromate battery is now used extensively. The solution may be made by dissolving one and a-half ounces of potassium bi chromate and two drachms of bi-sulphate of mercury in ten ounces of water, and slowly adding an ounce of sulphuric acid.

Ordinary battery fluid consists of one ounce of sulphuric acid in about ten ounces of water. To amalgamate a zinc plate, first immerse it in sulphuric acid and then in a bath of quicksilver; or it may be thoroughly washed with sulphuric acid and then a few beads of quicksilver placed upon it and spread over its surfaces. The dry cell or chloride of silver batteries are intended to avoid the inconveniences of fluid. They have many points of excellence, but have not demonstrated their claim to superiority.

Faradic Battery.- When a wire conducting electricity is approached by another and parallel wire, a current will be instantly induced through the second wire, opposite in direction to that in the first wire, but in the same direction at the instant of removal. This fact has been utilized for the production of a series of rapid electrical shocks. Faradic batteries are constructed upon the following principle, and are in most common use: A coil of wire covered with silk is formed as though wound about a spool; a second coil, large enough to slip over the first, is likewise formed. The ends of the first (primary) coil are attached to a battery cell, and the ends of the second (secondary) coil are attached to wires for use. An iron rod is placed within the primary coil. An automatic interrupter, called a rheotome, on the principle of spring and attraction, causes innumerably rapid current interruptions. The current is decreased by placing a brass or copper tube over the rod, or over the secondary coil, or between the two coils. Withdrawing the tube increases the current. Many Faradic batteries are constructed so that the galvanic current, direct from the cell, may be used separately.

Electro-Therapeutics.-The application of currents of electricity to the human body may produce stimulating, soothing or tonic effects. The molecular disturbances propagated through the molecules act remedially by causing contractions, exciting performances of function, helping elimination and the removal of obstructions, and aiding nutritive processes. The readiness with which such actions may be directed locally or generally by electricity, makes it especially valuable. It is most serviceable in chronic or sub-acute diseases; though for the relief of pain, or as a stimulant, or for its soothing action, it is frequently employed in acute cases. Like many other valuable agents, it was formerly, and by some still is regarded as a universal panacea. Its indiscriminate use by ignorant pretenders long kept it from receiving the professional attention which is now establishing its legitimate character as a therapeutical agent.

DIFFERENCES OF CURRENTS.

Galvanic currents are known as primary, direct, constant, voltaic, continuous or uninterrupted. Faradic are known as secondary, induced, inductive. to-and fro, interrupted, vibratory, magneto-electric or electro-magnetic.

The Galvanic current causes burning or stinging sensations, and easily produces chemical effects. It is regarded as relatively stronger than the Faradic, and superior for affecting deep seated structures. It is usually preferred in the treatment of neuralgia, rheumatism, persistent paralysis, atrophy, chronic diseases of the spinal cord, brain and sympathetic system, affections of the middle and internal ear, and for promoting alterations of the blood and aiding nutrition through nervous action. The galvanic current is almost universally employed for hastening absorption, discussing tumors and causing chemical destruction of substances. It is also most serviceable in causing evacuations of weakened vessels, and is employed in stoppage of the bowels and invagination; and is useful in exciting the performance of functions which have been disturbed by abnormal conditions of the muscles controlling them. It should be employed cautiously upon sensitive persons.

The Faradic current causes stinging and pricking sensations. It can be more easily endured than the galvanic, and in most cases should be employed first. It does not easily produce dizziness or unpleasant symptoms, and is safest for beginners. Its tonic action and its effects upon nutrition are most valuable. The thousands of rapid interruptions of the current during a sitting, cause a corresponding number of rapid contractions of the muscles and fibre cells resembling passive exercise. It is especially valuable in diseases of the abdominal viscera, and for promoting nutrition through muscular action. It should be employed when muscular contractions are desired when the muscles are not too much diseased to respond, as in early paralysis and general muscular debility. It is appropriate in acute affections of the brain and nervous system and in anaesthesia. Many eases are treated by alternating the galvanic and faradic currents. Most batteries are arranged for either, and a few for the simultaneous use of both currents, known as galvano-faradization.

DIFFERENCES OF POLES.

When held in the hands the negative pole gives the more decided electrical sensation, and is more painful than the positive.

When the electrodes of the two poles are placed an inch or so apart upon blotting paper saturated with solution of potassium iodide, a brown stain will be made by the positive. Blue litmus paper will be turned red by the positive, and red litmus paper will be turned blue by the negative electrode.

Uses.-As a convenient guide, the current from the positive pole may be figuratively regarded as "the pursuer," and the current from the negative pole as "the resister." The chief force of the current will be experienced near the negative pole, and in most cases that pole should be placed where irritation can be best endured, and the positive applied to sensitive structures; but no absolute rule can be formulated in this connection. When it is desired to break up adhesions or cause pronounced disturbances. the negative pole should be applied to the part. Astringent properties are attributed to the positive, making it useful to apply it to congestions, ulcerations and hemorrhages due to relaxed conditions; and the negative is applied to soften and produce relaxation. The positive pole is often spoken of as the anode, and the negative as the cathode.

TIME OF APPLICATION.

Bearing in mind that electricity causes molecular disturbances in structures, good judgment will dictate precautions against abuse. Damage may result from too free application, just as harm comes from excessive exercise or nervous strain. In most cases, mild currents of long duration are more beneficial than strong currents of short duration; though occasionally in obtuse subjects, the reverse of this is true. A desire to impress the patient with the power of the agent may result in absolute damage, where an almost imperceptible application would be of material benefit.

Daily applications of five, ten or fifteen minutes' duration may be regarded as a reasonable maximum use of electricity in chronic cases. Beginners and sensitive persons should be treated but every third or fourth day; though paralytics and some others may endure twenty-minute applications daily. General electrization should not be more frequent than once a week, as time should be allowed for reactive effects before additional disturbances are caused. Regularity as to the hour of electrical administration is unimportant unless particular effects are desired. Applications after the midday meal are often beneficial in atonic dyspepsia. For restlessness and insomnia, a mild Faradic current at the time of retiring will be found soothing. The system may become accustomed to electrical influences and require one or two weeks of rest. Some persons cannot endure electrization in any form, and others may endure strong currents without apparent effect. The age, sex and temperament must be considered, as well as the patient's feelings.

The beneficial use of electricity may be made manifest by inclination of the pulse and temperature toward the normal, lessening of pain, sense of mental exhilaration, soothing influence and pleasant drowsiness. Like other physical agents, such as heat and cold, electricity injudiciously applied may produce injurious effects.

Evidences of improper use may include headache, backache, sense of fatigue, soreness and aching, buzzing sounds, disturbances of vision, increase of pain and of pulse rate, irritability and excessive perspiration. Precautions must be taken against causing the slow-healing ulcers of the skin made possible by too frequent and prolonged applications of the electrode at any one spot. Injurious effects of electricity cannot be called toxic, as they are entirely physical.

General Faradization is a diffusive application of electricity throughout the body. Beneath the feet is placed a copper plate attached to the negative electrode, or the patient may sit upon the plate; a moistened sponge attached to the positive pole is slowly moved over the surface of the body. Sittings should seldom last over fifteen minutes, least time being given to the head and longest time to the spine.

Central Galvanization is occasionally employed to affect the central nervous system, especially when the exact seat of the disease is obscure, as in hysteria, chorea, hypochondria, etc. The negative electrode of a galvanic current is placed upon the epigastrium, and the positive is passed over the head, neck and spine. Cataphoresis is receiving considerable attention at the present time. It is based upon the principle that transfusions of liquids through porous substances are hastened by the electric current; thus the absorption of outward applications of medicinal solutions may be aided by applying the positive electrode.

Electrolysis is the decomposition of substance by electricity. Moles, warts, tumors and various growths may be thus destroyed. At least a twelve-celled, zinc-carbon-bichromate battery should be used. Gold, gold-plated, platinum, or iridio-platinum needles, attached to the negative pole, arc plunged into the growth and the positive electrode placed elsewhere. Superfluous hairs are removed by placing a single bulb-pointed needle beside the follicle and extracting the hair with small forceps when white froth appears at the root. Hemorrhoids, not inflamed, may be destroyed by seizing them with small forceps attached to the positive pole and plunging the negative needles into the tumors. Within five minutes they will turn white and be destroyed. Antiseptics should be employed. Bipolar electrodes, containing both poles close together, separated by an insulating septum, are of value for producing local effects within cavities, such as the bladder, uterus, vagina, urethra and rectum.

Static Electricity is generated by friction. For using it, modifications of the Holtz Machine, an expensive apparatus, are usually employed. Its administration requires insulation of the patient, and is termed Franklinization. Its employment is becoming more general, and its advantages and disadvantages better ascertained. A great variety of batteries and innumerable instruments have been invented for medical use, which can not be described here. Likewise space does not permit mention of the varied methods of applying electricity to meet the requirements of individual cases and special diseases. Guided by a knowledge of electro-therapeutics, the thoughtful physician will be able to harmonilze the use of electricity with other forms of treatment in a most successful manner.-WM. WESLEY COOK, M. D.

ELIXIRS.

An elixir as now understood in our pharmacy, is a form of syrup in which the bitter taste of drugs has been more or less effectually concealed by the skillful use of aromatics. We all like our doses to he as palatable as possible; and the day has gone by when the value of a remedy is estimated by its bitterness, and when a powder of hiera piera is a coveted morning potion. Some aromatics form good pharmacal combinations, others can not be associated to advantage; and some drugs can have their objectionable taste largely covered by a particular line of aromatics and adjuvants, while the same addenda would not be so effective with other drugs. It calls for much skill in the pharmacist to prepare suitable combinations by his art.

In attempting to make their preparations palatable, the essential feature of therapeutical efficiency has too often been lost sight of. Aromatics have been mingled and drugs left out till the product bas been rendered little more than a syrup of grateful flavor. Upon the patient such an elixir accomplishes nothing. In far too many instances manufacturing houses offer lists of this class of preparations, in each of which given amounts of certain drugs are said to be incorporated, whereas no such amounts of the medicaments could by any possibility be therein concealed.

This deception by the manufacturers is a most unworthy one toward the medical profession; and it has been carried so far by some houses as to have brought the entire class of elixirs into disfavor as being unreliable. But there are some preparations of this class that are at once desirable and reliable; and of these a few will be given here.

Simple Elixir, also called Elixir of Orange and Elixir Aurantii. This was introduced to the U. S. Pharmacopoeia that it might be an officinal preparation or base to which tinctures or fluid extracts could be added. It is an elegant vehicle for such purposes, made thus: Two and a half fluid drachms oil of orange are added, small portions at a time, to half an ounce of cotton, picking the cotton apart at each addition so as to distribute the oil thoroughly. The cotton is then packed tightly in a conical percolator, and a mixture of one pint of alcohol and two and a-half pints of water added gradually until three and a-quarter pints have passed through. To this add twenty-five ounces of granulated sugar, and dissolve by shaking and without heat. Strain.

Elixir of Beef, Wine and lron.-In an ounce and a half of distilled water dissolve 256 grains of ammonio citrate of iron. In fourteen and a half ounces of sherry wine dissolve half an ounce of Liebig's extract of beef, and add half an ounce spirit of orange (1 to 10), mix the two. This is commonly spoken of as Beef, Wine and Iron; and is entirely overrated as a tonic. It is little better than an excuse for prescribing wine.

Elixir of Calisaya.-Triturate into a pint of the simple elixir 72 grains sulphate quinine, 24 grains sulphate cinchonine, 20 grains sulphate quinidine, 12 grains sulphate cinchonidine. Put into a glass flask and heat on a water bath till the whole is dissolved. Add to this, while hot, 7 pints simple elixir and enough caramel to color. When cold, filter.

It is frequently desirable to get the virtues of an agent free from its tannic acid. This is readily accomplished by first obtaining a tincture of the agent with such strength of an alcoholic menstruum as is advisable; have ready a solution of the hydrated oxide of iron to which one-fourth part of alcohol has been added; and add this to the tincture of the article till its tannic acid has been occupied by the iron and deposited. The complete removal of the tannin is determined by adding a drop of tincture of chloride of iron to a portion of the filtered article, which will give no coloration if all the tannin has been removed. An article thus deprived of its tannic acid is said to be detannated. Cinchona, prunus cornus, and some other remedies containing tannic acid, are sometimes detannated; and such a preparation is then miscible with iron solutions without causing an inky discoloration and deposit.

Elixir Calisaya Bark.-This is an elegant detannated elixir of Peruvian bark, in many respects preferable to the above elixir of the cinchona salts. In quantities of five gallons, it is prepared as follows: Calisaya bark 24 ounces, orange peel 16, coriander 4, cinnamon 3, cardamom 1 1/2, anise 1, cocoa (Baker's) 8, troy weight. Suitably ground, this mixture is treated in the percolator by 1 measure of alcohol and 3 measures of water till 2I gallons have passed. This is detannated as above, and then strained through muslin, and finally enough of the menstruum passed through the residue on the strainer to make the whole measure 5 gallons. To this is added half an ounce of oil of orange triturated with 6 ounces precipitated chalk, the whole thoroughly mixed, and finally filtered through paper. Dissolve in this 15 pounds of sugar.

Elixir Calisaya and lron.-To 16 fluid ounces of either of the above calisaya elixirs add 256 grains citrate of iron and ammonia, or citrate of iron and potassa. Many elixirs are made by adding to the simple elixir from 1 to 3 fluid ounces of the fluid extracts of the medicaments employed, first adding to them 2 fluid ounces of alcohol, and filtering; the whole to make one pint.

Elixir Glycyrrhiza.-In 6 fluid ounces of alcohol put 5 drops oil of cloves and 3 drops oil of cinnamon; add this to half a pint of simple syrup and 2 ounces fluid extract licorice, shake well with a drachm of carbonate magnesia, filter through muslin. This elixir is much used to conceal the taste of quinine.

EMBELIA RIBES.

From Hindostan, and especially from the province of Bombay, the fruit of this immense climbing shrub has come. It is a berry resembling black pepper, of a moderately bitter and slightly aromatic taste. Among the inhabitants of the Indies these berries are employed for the removal of the tapeworm, from a drachm to half an ounce or more of their powder being given in milk early in the morning. A dose of castor oil precedes and follows the medicine. It is said to expel the entire worm, dead; and as it is an article quite acceptable to the stomach, it naturally has become very popular in a country where taenia flourishes to such an extent that every third person is said to be afflicted with it. It is also reputed useful in flatulent dyspepsia, and as an alterative in skin disease.

A principle called embelic acid has been obtained from this fruit. It comes in crystalline scales of a dull orange color, without taste or odor. Neutralized with ammonia and dried, it forms the salt ammonium embelicum; and the dose of this for children is from 2 to 3 grains, for an adult 6 to 7 grains, fasting. Some physicians consider it a more reliable tamiacide than male fern or pomegranate.

EPHEDRA ANTISYPHILITICA.

MOUNTAIN RUSH, MORMON TEA.

Western Texas, Nevada, Utah, and portions of California abound in this low, shrubby plant. Considerable quantities of a reddish-brown resin exist in its medullary portion. This resin possesses both stimulating and astringing properties, which act on the mucous tissues and the glandular system. It is a people's remedy for gonorrhoea and similar diseases of the genital passages; and for stimulating and depurating the system in constitutional syphilis. It is of no small activity, and evidently deserves professional attention; and probably will be found useful in various skin diseases of constitutional origin.

EQUISETUM HYEMALE.

SCOURING RUSH, SHAVE GRASS, HORSETAIL.

Along the brooks ides and other wet places, especially in the Northward, this rush is common, its rough and slender stem growing to a height of from 18 inches to 2 feet.

Housewives use it for scouring purposes, its silica being finer and sharper than the famous sapolio. From time to time it has been mentioned as a diuretic, and then dismissed from attention. It deserves more consideration; for it possesses stimulating with astringing properties, and expends its power on the kidneys and urinary passages in a desirable manner. It increases the flow of urine moderately, aiding in the general elimination of the renal solids without exhausting the kidneys, but rather leaving behind a goodly tonic impression. Such qualities are desirable in many cases of dropsy, congestion of the kidneys with diminution of their function, haematuria, and similar troubles. In gleet the article often answers a good purpose; and at times it has been spoken of for gravel, probably from its influence in increasing the renal flow. I have also used it in some cases of prolapsus with leucorrheoa and persistent backache, and believe it deserves to be studied in this connection. The profession will be advantaged by getting acquainted with this agent. Used by infusion, or 20 to 30 drops of fluid extract.

ERIODICTYON GLUTINOSUM.

YERBA SANTA, MOUNTAIN BALM, BEAR'S WEED.

Upon the dry hills of California this little shrub grows abundantly. Its leaves are lanceolate, 3 to 6 inches long, thick, and of a somewhat leathery texture, having a resinous feel, smooth above, white with a fine wooliness underneath. The leaves are the medicinal portion, and contain 30 percent or more of a gum resin, a small amount of volatile oil, and some tannin.

Medical Properties.- Yerba Santa (the Holy Herb) was long used by the Spaniards of California and Mexico before it came to professional notice; and the name they gave it suggests the esteem in which it was held by them. In 1873, a friend sent me some of the leaves; and I at once apprehended their character and proceeded to use them with great satisfaction, but had no specimens to enable me to give them their botanical place. A few years later Dr. J. H. Bundy attracted earnest attention to it, and the house of Parke, Davis & Co. aided materially in enlisting the profession toward it.

It is a stimulant with some relaxant properties, of the gum resinous or balsamic class, leaving behind a slightly tonic impression. Its action is moderately prompt and rather persistent; and, like many other balsams, is largely expended on the bronchial mucous surfaces, and on the renal organs and pelvic mucosa to a fair degree. It is most efficacious in bronchial affections, especially in sub-acute and chronic inflammations with severe and spasmodic cough, tickling, scanty and tenacious expectoration, and asthmatic breathing. In all such troubles it is of signal efficacy, securing freer expectoration without relaxing the parts, and affording prompt relief. Among such conditions come bronchorrhoea and the distressing winter cough of elderly persons. Laryngeal congestions are equally amenable to it. Some have commended it in whooping-cough; but I have not found it of much service there, although it makes a suitable addition to castanea when a stimulating expectorant is advisable in the advanced stages. In asthma, it is beneficial by hastening the expulsion of the tenacious mucus, and affords much relief to many cases; and a little lobelia with it makes an effective combination. Smoking the leaves in asthma is a common practice among the natives. Being itself largely stimulating, it may be combined with the relaxing glycyrrhiza, especially when it is necessary to allay the vexatious tickling in the throat that accompanies many coughs. In cases of phthisis, the yerba santa alone is good for throat tickling; but beyond its influence as a reliable balsamic expectorant, it is not to be depended on in that malady. For chronic coughs with weakness of the respiratory mucous membranes and profuse expectoration, its stimulating and mildly tonic properties make it an admirable article, especially if aided by the antispasmodic and astringent properties of either of the viburnums of hamamelis, or of trillium. In aphonia, and the half-paralyzed condition of the laryngeal muscles of some coughs, it is excellent, alone or with such a stimulant as xanthoxylum. The action of yerba santa on the renal organs deserves more attention than it has received, especially in chronic cystitis and gleet. It makes a fair stimulating addendum to such diuretics as eupatorium purpureum and juniper berries; and to such uterine agents as mitchella and polygonatum for lax conditions of the female organs. Dose of the fluid extract, 5 to 30 drops or more every four or three hours. Its resinous character prevents its being miscible with water; but when a little alkali is added it is more miscible and makes a clear mixture with syrups. Combined with coriander, cinnamon and other aromatics it is used to disguise the bitterness of quinine. It is not compatible with acids.

EUCALYPTUS GLOBULUS.

GUM TREE, BLUE GUM, FEVER TREE.

Eucalyptus is a native of Australia, where it is an immense tree with large, thick, and somewhat glossy leaves, a bluish-gray bark, and a pale, heavy and durable wood. Its leaves are the medicinal portion, and contain a strongly odorous volatile oil, different resins, and tannin. The oil is the element on which its remedial qualities depend; and that which passes over at the lower degrees of heat is the most valuable, being also the most abundant. It is a light-brown fluid, of a peculiar and penetrating odor, and. on redistillation from caustic potash furnishes the clear, white and thin eucalyptol. Other species of the genus eucalyptus are said not to furnish eucalyptol, or to yield it only in minute quantities.

This tree was reputed to be capable of neutralizing the miasmatic poison, and to free malarial district" from the miasmatic dangers. It hence was cultivated in large sections of southern Europe and America, where it is now abundant. Probably its wonderfully rapid growth and the immense size of its numerous leaves, which are often a foot in length, use up the moistness of the marshy grounds, and thus arrest the paludal dangers. Its efficiency in thus preventing the vegetable decay from which the germs of malaria arise, has been well attested; and to this, rather than to the influence of its exhalations, are to be attributed its virtues in rendering habitable certain large district formerly ravaged by malaria.

Medical Properties. -Eucalyptus leaves are stimulating, prompt and rather diffusive in action, penetrating and tenacious in their impression, having an aromatic and somewhat balsamic odor and character all its own. Whether the leaves or any preparation from them is med, it gives a pungent and warming impression on the tongue, fauces and stomach, which soon extend through the lungs, the entire respiratory tract being influenced by the agent. On this account it is employed in congestion and low grades of inflammation of the fauces, larynx and bronchi. An antiseptic power is associated with it, as with most balsams and volatile oils. Its influence in this respect, . however, is due largely to its stimulating action on the arterioles and arterial capillaries; for as a germicide its power is but as 1 to 88, whereas boracic acid is 1 to 140, benzoic acid 1 to 900, and essence of cinnamon 1 to 3,000. But even this feeble germicidal power, coupled with its positive stimulating action on mucous membranes, renders it a valuable agent in purulent, degenerate and fetid discharges from the throat, lungs, vagina, etc. Hence it has been found of peculiar service in diphtheria, gangrene and foul abscesses of the lungs, purulent bronchitis, offensive leucorrhea, putrid dysentery, and similar maladies. Taken by the stomach, it is soon absorbed and its peculiar odor noticed in the breath. It was thought that eucalyptus would prove a strong anti-periodic, but this has not been verified, although many use it freely in malarial diseases. Results are not uniform, and the benefits from it are indirect, from its diffusively stimulating power. Lately it has obtained prominence as an intestinal stimulant and antiseptic in typhoid fever, small doses being given at moderate intervals; and if the reports in its favor should be verified by further experience, it will prove a desirable agent here. Malignant scarlatina is said to be rendered much less serious by its antiseptic power; and from the promptness with which it is absorbed, it is used in cases of pyoomia, whether in gynocological or surgical practice, outwardly upon degenerate ulcers and cancers.
A powerful agent, covering a peculiar and very large field of usefulness, it has been natural for its employment and praises to be carried to an extreme. Give it its right position as a stimulant and fair antiseptic of balsamic character, and it can be used intelligently. There are some reports showing that excessive doses, after first exciting the cerebral circulation and causing headache, afterwards induced vaso-motor depression through the spinal cord, with pallor, cold extremities and prostration. These facts deserve careful and anxious consideration.

Eucalyptus oil is the essential constituent, and is given in doses of 2 to 10 drops, three or four hours apart. Larger quantities have been used, but are not desirable. It may be given in capsule, combined with almond oil, or as an emulsion. A fluid extract is prepared, and is given by emulsion in doses of 5 to 20 drops. A powdered solid extract, in doses of 2 to 5 grains, rubbed in lactin, is preferred by some. For diphtheria, ozoena, foetid bronchitis, and similar conditions, it is best used as an inhalant, the refined eucalyptol being mingled with a neutral oil. Such inhalations are suitable in many cases of chronic bronchitis and pulmonary cavities; but there is no reliable evidence of eucalyptus having any direct effect upon tuberculosis. My own favorite inhalant for respiratory troubles is eucalyptol in benzoinol. A proprietary medicine by Bracelin seems a mixture of eucalyptol, thymol and menthol, the alleged chlorine being a myth; the combination being an inhalant of considerable antiseptic and stimulating power, and a good adjunct to other treatment in diphtheria. For vaginal use euca]yptol is much diluted with oil, and applied by cotton plug or in suppositories.

Eucalyptus Rostrata, known as Red Gum, is another of the family belonging to Australia. Upon its bark is a red-colored exudation of a gummy character, and nearly all soluble in water. It is an active astringent, soothing and leaving a goodly tonic impression. In many respects it resembles the kino; and like the latter it reduces mucous discharges without so astringing the tissue as to leave undue deficiency of secretion. It has an advantage over kino in not forming an insoluble semi-gelatinous mass when its tincture gets old. It is used in the same classes of cases as most other astringents.

EUGENIA CHEQUEN.

CHEKAN.

Allied to the myrtus, and frequently classed as myrtus chekan. A plant native to Chili, growing into a small tree along the sandy river beds, but dwarfing to a low shrub on the uplands. The leaves contain an agreeable volatile oil as their chief medicinal ingredient, with a small amount of a bitter principle and some tannin. The fluid extract put upon the market is made from the leaves.

Medical Properties.-Chekan is a stimulant, with some tonic qualities, almost balsamic, acting well upon the mucous surfaces. Its chief influence is upon the bronchial passages; but it also acts on the intestinal and vaginal surfaces, and quite favorably upon the kidneys. It is suited to relaxed and feeble conditions of these surfaces; hence its marked usefulness in the winter cough of elderly people, and in chronic bronchitis with purulent expectoration. In all such troublesome conditions it loosens the tenacious expectoration, abates the cough, removes the purulent characters of the sputum and gives much relief to the general distress. Even in advanced phthisis it often proves of service as a sustaining expectorant, where it is too often the plan to use weakening relaxants. In corresponding states of the genitalia with semi-purulent leucorrhoea, it is good locally and by the stomach. Dose, half a fluid drachm to two drachms every three or four hours.

EUGENIA JAMBOLANA.

JAMBUL.

Also called syzygium jambolanum. Another member of the Myrtus or Chekan family; a goodly tree abounding in the East Indies in a wild state, and much cultivated for its edible fruit.

Medical Properties.-An astringent property, due to gallic acid, is found in the bark and leaves, which are used by the natives in various washes, gargles, and other preparations where an astringent is needed. It is now claimed that the seeds, and in a smaller measure the hark, arrest the formation of sugar, and hence arc useful in diabetes. They are stimulating to the spinal cord, influencing its reflex and vaso-motor functions, and thus reaching the heart and increasing its activity and force. Such properties are desirable in a strictly non-toxic agent, and make it a suitable remedy in various nerve depressions and exhaustions; and jambul has shown promising qualities in languor, crampings, night-sweats, etc. Used in diabetes mellitus it soon and notably diminishes the amount of urine and the percentage of sugar, relieves the thirst, improves the condition, heals up diabetic ulcers, and restores the patient. Such are the reports of some medical observers.

It would seem to be adapted to diabetes of nervous origin, where so many of our familiar nervines, as viburnum opulus, celastrus, scutellaria, and others, have so often proven efficient. The agent, as well as the pathology of the malady, needs careful investigation. Dose of the powdered seeds, 5 to 10 grains three times a day; the same in drops of fluid extract.

EUPATORIUM PURPUREUM.

QUEEN-OF-THE-MEADOW, GRAVEL ROOT.

Several other plants have received the common name of gravel root. because of their action on the kidneys; the epigea repens and liatris spicata being instances. The article here under consideration is a member of the boneset tribe; and has long been employed for its excellent relaxant and soothing influence on the kidneys, bladder and urethra, increasing the flow of urine and allaymg irritation. It has a similar beneficial action on the female genitalia, making a serviceable addition to other agents in gynecological practice.

In 1876 I published my observations on the influence of this remedy on the spinal cord and the prostate gland; and continued experience has more than confirmed the views I then offered. It exerts a peculiar and mild, but persistent and reliable influence on the cord and its meninges, extending its impressions to the nerves of the entire genito-urinary apparatus.

Being relaxant, it is not suited to depressed and enfeebled conditions; but to states of sensitiveness, tenderness and irritability. In that condition known as spinal irritation, a frequent clinical fact though sometimes disputed by pathologists, this eupatorium is excellent. Under its mild action, the spinal tenderness gradually abates, and a relief from suffering is obtained that I have never been able to secure from any other agent. It also relieves the spinal tenderness and aching reflex from uterine and ovarian troubles, soothing the latter organs in a desirable manner.

Its influence on the female sexual organs makes it useful in hysteria, sub-acute metritis and endometritis, ovarian tenderness, etc. Upon the prostate it acts quite decidedly, and is of great service in prostatic suffering and enlargement, and in certain forms of irritable spermatorrhoea. So few agents influence this gland, that this quality of eupatorium purpureum is desirable and valuable. Being in itself so largely relaxant, it is often well to combine it with agents of a different class. In spinal erethism, my favorite course has been to associate it with leaves of amygdalus, and usually a limited portion of viburnum opulus also. For vesical troubles, the epigea repens, in a moderate quantity, is a suitable synergist; and for spermatorrhoea it may be combined with flowers of althea rosea and a small portion of hydrastis. Dose of fluid extract, 20 to 60 drops every 3 hours.

FEHROM.

IRON AND ITS COMPOUNDS.

Iron has been used as a medicine from the earliest times, dating as a remedy from the period when minerals in general were believed to be the best curative agencies. As iron was the most abundant and the most useful of metals, it was an easy step in ancient logic to conclude that the gods had endowed it with the strongest remedial powers. In more recent periods that mode of reasoning has been laid aside, and iron has been employed on the basis of its being I't component of the red corpuscles of the blood; and hence it was concluded that it would multiply and invigorate the corpuscles when these were deficient and the blood was" thin. "

The total amount of iron in the human body is so very small, that if all the metal in a ferric preparation were actually put into the corpuscles, a few doses would furnish all the metal that the blood could contain normally. It is, however, by no means determined that iron as a medicine is absorbed, though it has long been believed that such is the physiological method of appropriating it. Recent, and more accurate investigations have shown that the iron given as medicine is itself excreted; and while the uniform presence of this metal in the blood intimates its necessity, the small amount required is furnished by the organic substances used as food, and not by presenting iron in an inorganic form. That a very small portion may be taken up into the system is possible, though even that has not been shown to full satisfaction; but if it is, there is no evidence to sustain the idea that it is assimilated into the red corpuscles, but rather that it is separated and expelled by way of the portal circulation and the liver.

It seems altogether most probable that iron and its compounds are acted on, chemically, by the sulphur gases that exist in the upper portion of the alimentary canal under many circumstances. Such gases are common in health when certain foods are used, and become abnormally abundant in anaemic conditions and other states where intestinal digestion is greatly at fault.

It seems probable that these sulphides have such a greed for iron as to rob the very food of this element, and thus create a deficiency in the supply furnished to the blood; hence the medicinal use of iron satisfies the demand of the sulphides and leaves the assimilative organs to obtain that element from the organic supply in the food the offensive and detrimental character of the sulphides being overcome, the iron sulphides thus formed in the bowels are evacuated in the blackened feces. It is in this way that iron renders its first benefit to. the system.

Apart from the above action, iron and some of its preparations are slow stimulants to the intestinal and portal circulations, and may increase the force of the general circulation, on which latter account this element is not to be used when there is any exalted blood pressure, but rather when the heart force is reduced and the system lax. It improves intestinal digestion and promotes assimilation; and it is by these influences, rather than by in any degree supplying the red corpuscles with the iron element, that this article increases the richness of the blood and becomes a general tonic. Its usefulness is limited to the field above indicated, feeble intestinal digestion with laxity of structures, offensive flatulence, defective assimilation, anaemia and chlorosis with the peculiar train of symptoms connected with the various degrees of blood impoverishment.

As an aid to other medication, a suitable preparation of iron is unquestionably valuable in such conditions. It may then properly be termed a tonic; but not in the same sense that Hydrastis, colomba or cinchona is a tonic.

Iron preparations are best used near the times of eating. If they so arouse the circulation as to flush the face or cause headache, they should be discontinued. No vegetable astringent is compatible with any soluble iron preparation as the resultant chemical compound is a species of ink. Springs containing iron are known as chalybeate waters, and there are great numbers of these. The amount of iron in these waters is generally small; and being in soluble form it acts promptly and agreeably, whence the drinking of some good chalybeate water is an excellent way to obtain the tonic effects of iron.

Solution of sub-sulphate of iron (Monsell's solution) is one of the most effective styptics, coagulating the blood in bleeding vessels, and being less irritating than solution of the ter-sulphate.

Iron Chlorides, in solution or as tincture, are strongly astringent and styptic, and have an acid reaction from the presence of free hydrochloric acid. It has been supposed that this acid would assist the gastric juice; and so tincture of iron came to be used extensively as a tonic for indigestion, often combined with gentian and with detannated cinchona. It is a pleasant theory, but actual practice has shown that the presence of free hydrochloric acid, while tolerated for a time, finally denudes the stomach of its fine epithelium and causes chronic inflammation that is exceedingly intractable.

Ferrum Albuminatum, Albuminate of Iron, is prepared from an admixture of ferric sulphate with a solution of albumen, the precipitate being dissolved in an excess of alkali, and the alkali and the sulphuric acid removed by dialysis. The clear solution that remains contains the iron in conj unction with albumen, being a solution of a salt in which the acid of the sulphate is replaced by albumen. It is of neutral reaction, without metallic or astringent taste, not affected in its medical properties by the addition of alcohol, alkali, or an excess of acid, and keeps well. It contains, as put upon the market, one-half of one per cent. of iron oxide in a state of solution. This Liquor Ferri Albuminati is one of the most acceptable iron preparations to the stomach, acts promptly, and is among the more serviceable ferric preparations. Dose, 10 to 40 drops. Ferri et. Potassii Tartras, Tartrate of Iron and Potassium, is an old preparation having the advantages of being a neutral salt that is very soluble in water. It is, therefore, free from all acid and styptic qualities, is not astringent, is pleasant to the taste and acceptable to the stomach. Should it be true that iron accomplishes a portion of benefit by being absorbed, then this preparation from its lack of astringency is one of the most absorbable ferric compounds. It may be given in doses of ten to twenty grains, in water or syrup, three times a day; but I have been best pleased when giving but two to three grains as a dose. My favorite mode of exhibiting it is with hydrastia phosphate, in syrup zingiher, as a stomachic and intestinal tonic compound, taken half an hour to an hour after meals. A minute quantity tincture of myrrh may be added to arrest fermenta.tive processes. Ammonia-tartrate of iron is similar. Ferrum Sanguinis, or Iron of the Blood, has been put upon the market by different manufacturers and under different names. It has been supposed that, if obtained from the blood of animals, iron would be more assimilable because of its derivation from an organic source. It should be remembered, however, that when a metallic element has been separated from an organic compound into which it has entered, the organized character of that compound has been broken up by chemical processes, and the isolated mineral stands alone again. The claim of greater assimilability for iron derived from blood, has not been sustained to the satisfaction of all observers; and there is a growing opinion that the zeal of commercial competition has too often covered up therapeutical exactness.

This opinion is strengthened when each new product under the class of Ferrum Sanguinis is promoted by evidence that the products of other manufacturers in the same class have proven unassimilable. It remains true of them all that iron which has been isolated from the blood no longer possesses organic qualities, but each such product must be judged by its own action on the system. HAEMOGALLOL is another ferruginous blood preparation. Dose, 3 to 8 grains.

Among the iron preparations of this class are Haemoglobin and Ferratin. The latter was first obtained from the blood of the liver; but is now made up synthetically, and is therefore an artificial product. These and others in the class Ferrum Sanguinis are mostly non-astringent, neutral, well received by the stomach, and hence quite advantageous under many circumstances.

FERULA SUMBUL.

MUSK ROOT, SUMBUL.

A perennial herb of central Asia, the spongy root of which is used in medicine. It contains a resinous substance, and has a rather pronounced and not unpleasant musk-like odor, which is persistent. Its taste is aromatic and rather bitter.

Medical Properties.-Musk root is a prompt and diffusive relaxant and stimulant, somewhat transient in its effects. Such properties render it antispasmodic; and the agent is effective in relieving spasmodic and nervous troubles that require a soothing and sustaining influence on the spinal reflexes. Hence, it becomes useful in all hysterical manifestations, and in general nervous agitations; while the uterine organs and nervous system are being toned by such agents as polygonatum, viburnum and caulophyllum. Russian physicians have employed it in cholera, but I cannot see that it has any direct relation to the pathology of that malady. It has been spoken of in epilepsy, as have so many other antispasmodics. In my judgment the article deserves close investigation. Dose, 2 to 5 drops every four or two hours.

FRANKENIA GRANDIFLORA.

YERBA REUMA, FLUX HERB.

A small shrub native to California. It contains a considerable percentage of tannin, a large amount of an acid resin. and a notable amount of soda sulphate and chloride. It is used chiefly for the astringing tonic properties of its leaves, which have. been well spoken of as a local application in leucorrhoea, catarrh, gleet, and other places where such an agent is needed, and internally for chronic dysentery and diarrhoea. Dose of fluid extract, 5 to 15 drops, largely diluted.

FUCUS VESICULOSUS.

BLADDER-WRACK, SEA-WRACK.

Among inhabitants of the sea shores in Europe this seaweed has long been held in esteem for the treatment of goiter and scrofulous swellings. Latterly it has been observed to have the power of reducing the amount of fat in the system, and has acquired a wide reputation in this connection. In what manner it effects this is not well determined; but it seems to act upon the entire lymphatic and absorbent systems, distinctly altering the assimilative processes and promoting the deposit of muscular fibre while reducing the redundant adipose tissue. M. Duchesne-Dupare discovered these qualities of the article. It appears to be chiefly relaxant in action, with a moderate stimulating effect, and a peculiar and not always acceptable taste. Dr. Griffith, in his essay on corpulence, says: " After using it some time the patient feels lighter and more active; the stomach acts with more rapidity, flatulence disappears, and digestion is no longer accompanied by flushings and weight in the epigastrium, and flashes of heat toward the head." It has been found to promote absorption in some dropsies, cervical deposits, etc. It increases urination after being used three or four weeks, and then the reduction of fat begins and will continue steadily. Its action is aided by full catharsis, and by reduction of farinaceous and fatty foods. Improving the general health by removing abnormal obesity, it will be accompanied by improved menstruation and digestion; and it is of benefit in chronic cystitis. In fluid extract form, half a drachm to two drachms may be given three times a day. Some prefer it in decoction, drank freely. No functional disturbances follow its free use.

GARCINIA MANGOSTANA.

MANGOSTEEN.

A tree of medium size, native to the Malay archipelago and adjacent lands, bearing a delicate edible fruit about the size of an apple. The pericarp of this fruit is medicinal.

Medical Properties.-Mangosteen is a tonic of the astringent class, and imparts firmness and vigor to mucous membranes without constipating, in which it resembles the tonic astringency of gum kino. It seems to possess a fair measure of stimulation. For chronic diarrhma it is good; but for uterine hemorrhages, profuse menstruation, and the excessive wastes that often follow miscarriage, it is valuable. Upon tbe uterus it exerts a most excellent effect, closely resembling that of viburnum prunifolium but stronger.

Some physicians have spoken highly of it as a local application in diphtheria and other degenerate laryngal affections, in foul leucorrhma, cervical erosions, purulent discharges and offensive sores. Dose, 5 to 20 drops, repeated as indicated.

GARRYA FREMONTII.

CALIFORNIA FEVER BUSH.

A member of the Cornaceae or Dogwood family, native to California, where it is a beautiful evergreen shrub 5 to 8 feet high, with leathery oblong leaves one to three inches in length. Its leaves are intensely bitter, and quite persistent in action.

Medical Properties.-From the early days of the occupancy of California by Americans, the leaves of this plant have been used by them as a tonic. They are stimulatmg, influencing the stomach, the glandular system, circulation, and probably the spinal nerves. They give a sense of warmth in the epigastrium, arouse the pulse, send the blood freely to the brain, and moderately increase the general secretions. Their principal use has been as a tonic against intermittents, being given between the paroxysms as cinchona and its salts are given, and are warmly commended by a number of physicians as very reliable. Over cinchona they possess an advantage in not being astringent, opening up the emunctories instead of closing them. This property makes garrya of service in atonic conditions of the stomach; and gives it a wide field of usefulness in many conditions of debility, in convalescence, and as a tonic adjuvant to other remedies in scrofula and amenorrhea. Dose, 5 to 20 or more drops of the liquid extract, repeated according to indications.

GLYCERINUM.

GLYCERINE.

Glycerine, obtained by decomposing fixed oils and animal fats, has become a necessity to the physician; although experience has shown that the place first given to it in therapeutics could not be sustained. As a remedy in phthisis it has proven a failure; but it is a suitable adjunct in mixtures for recent and irritable coughs, where glycerine one part and mucilage of acacia two parts may be employed as a menstruum for fluid extracts of glycyrrhiza, prunus, and similar agents. Its fair antiseptic properties make it a suitable addition to sprays intended for diphtheria, catarrh, and other throat and nasal troubles. It also assists in retaining the medicament~ upon the parts when thus used. Its continued use in any considerable quantities to the stomach is not favorable to good digestion; and a four-ounce mixture of any preparation for internal use should not contain more than three drachms of glycerine.

Outwardly it is an agent of much value in cases where an emollient is needed. Having a strong affinity for water, it cannot be used alone without inviting to itself the fluids of the capillaries and causing an unpleasant stinging sensation. This is very unpleasant and objectionable if pure glycerine is applied to a mucous surface, as to the vagina. On this account glycerine is mixed with from two to four times its own bulk of water when employed externally; and the soothing property of rosewater makes it serviceable for these purposes. Such mixtures are popular for roughness and chapping of the skin; and for scaly cutaneous diseases with inflammation, as prurigo, psoriasis, herpes, eczema, etc. Suitable medicaments may be added to glycerine and water as a wash for such purposes, among which hydrastis, liquid hydrastis and distilled hamamelis may be mentioned. For crusting herpes and eczema I have been in the habit of applying one drachm fluid extract hydrastis in two ounces each of glycerine and rose water, giving relief and effecting cures in old cases that had proven wholly intractable to the usual remedies. It obviates the use of lard, which is so objectionable in many skin diseases.

A small proportion of glycerine in poultices keeps them soft; and the same is effected by adding it to a pill mass. Various ointments are improved by an admixture with glycerine, mainly by an incorporation of it with spermaceti and white wax.

One of the best of these is made by melting together one ounce of spermaceti, three drachms of white wax, and four ounces oil of almonds; then adding one ounce and a half of glycerine and rubbing in a mortar till cold. A glycerine jelly is made by dissolving 70 parts white castile soap shavings in 105 parts of glycerine, and then gradually adding with rapid trituration 630 parts ojl sweet almonds, 4 parts oil bergamot and 1 part oil of rose. One-twentieth part of borax may be added to either of these preparations. One ounce of borax will dissolve in four fluid ounces of glycerine when rubbed in a mortar, constituting the glycerite of borax, and a much larger portion will dissolve by heat, forming the BORO-GLYCERIDE.

Both these preparations are excellent for aphthous sores and similar conditions, diluted as required, their sweetness making them acceptable to children and their antiseptic properties being desirable.

Glycerite of Tannic Acid (Glyceritum acidi tannici) is prepared by rubbing together one ounce of tannin and four fluid ounces glycerine and gently heating till the tannin is dissolved. It is a fine preparation whenever tannic acid is wanted locally. Glycerite of Starch (Glyceritum amyli) is made by rubbing together one ounce of starch and seven fluid ounces of glycerine, then heating gradually to 28° F., till the starch dissolves into a jelly. It is used as a pleasant demulcent locally, and a plasma with which to make poultices or mix powders. Messrs. Parke, Davis & Co. prepare a Glycerine Emollient, of gaultheria 2 parts, boric acid 23, starch 88, glycerine 885, tragacanth 17. It is designed to take the place of vaseline in gynecological practice, and is a fine emollient, antiseptic, deodorant and detergent.

Glycerine is also made into suppositories for laxative purposes. Fifty parts cocoa butter, 20 parts glycerine, 2 parts powdered tragacanth, make ten suppositories. Much larger percentages of glycerine may be incorporated with borax and a little tragacanth. They act quickly in emergencies, lubricating the rectum and provoking a watery discharge; but they are too sharp to be continued for any length of time, and will not cure chronic constipation. The late Dr. F. Marion Sims put glycerine to local use by wetting a tampon of cotton in water, squeezing it, and then mingling in the cotton It teaspoonful of glycerine and placing this up against the cervix. It depletes the overcharged blood vessels by inviting the water through their walls to the glycerine, thus securing a flow of water and giving material comfort to the congested vessels. This procedme frequently arrests the reflex vomiting of pregnaney.

Melted glue may be mixed with glycerine, the water almost entirely evaporated, any desired medicaments added to this, and the mass then moulded into suppositories. Such suppositories are flexible and melt at the warmth of the body.

Because of its softening and antiseptic action on the skin, glycerine enters into a large number of fluid and creamy toilet preparations and dentifrices. Much ingenuity has been exercised in getting up such mixtures, most of which contain one part of borax to 20 or 40 parts of glycerine and fragrant waters to suit the fancy.

GYNOCARDIA ODORATA.

CHAULMOOGRA.

Gynocardia is a large tree native to the Malayan peninsula. Its fruit is as large as an orange, and produces many large seeds. By expression, or by boiling the crushed seeds in water, they yield a fixed oil, of a pale or golden amber color, and a faint and somewhat unpleasant smell. It contains several acid principles, the most abundant being palmitic acid, and the characteristic one being gynocardic acid.

Chaulmoogra oil, and its active principle, gynocardic acid, are stimulating, of a slightly acrid taste, and not acceptable to an empty stomach. Large doses are emetic. The oil has long been popular among the natives as an outward application for stiff joints and sprains, rheumatism and neuralgia. It has come into professional use in eczema, psoriasis and other inflammatory skin diseases; an ointment of one part of oil and two of vaseline, or twenty grains of gynocardic acid to the ounce of vaseline, affording relief from the stinging and effecting a cure, used several times a day. It has been commended in lupus; and used both outwardly and inwardly in leprosy, and intractable secondary syphilis. Its inward use frequently disturbs the stomach, upsets the appetite, and brings on looseness of the bowels. It has been spoken of in phthisis, but has no merits in that relation. Dose of the oil, 2 to 4 drops three times a day; best given in capsule or emulsion.

HAMAMELIS VIRGINICA.

WITCH HAZEL.

After having been in use for a century, and suffering contempt at the hands of those who did not understand its value, this remedy has been" discovered" and become professionally popular. Its leaves are an admirable astringent of a medium grade, with some nervine and tonic properties.

Few agents act so kindly and reliably in contracting the walls of the venous capillaries; and while in no sense a haemostatic like ferrum sulphate, it is of great service in haematuria, passive menorrhagia, haemoptysis, and similar capillary bleedings. One of its finest uses is for anal fissure and bleeding piles, where it both soothes the suffering and arrests the bleeding; used as an ointment or in suppository and also given internally.

In vesical catarrh, leucorrhrna, aphthous sores, and similar conditions of the mucous membranes, it is a serviceable agent, especially when combined with hydrastis. I have used it successfully in four cases of chyluria.

For thirty years I contended that hamamelis contained a volatile principle. Finally this was obtained by distillation, and the elegant article, "distilled witch hazel, " is now common. It is used outwardly for bruises, muscular soreness, sprains, etc.; and inwardly as a wash for leucorrhrna, gleet, sore mouth, vesical catarrh, and similar conditions. It is an admirable article for all these purposes; and for inward use may be combined with one-fourth part liquid hydrastis.

A good ointment for haemorrhoids may be made of one drachm extract hamamelis, twenty grains powdered hydrastis, one ounce mutton tallow, and sufficient olive oil to soften.

HYDRANGEA ARBORESCENS.

SEVEN BARKS, WILD HYDRANGEA.

Our native hydrangea is a pretty shrub five or six feet high, with light green and broad leaves, and bunches of small white flowers that gradually become ruddy. Its bark peels off in a series of different colored layers. The shrub is abundant east, west and south, on rocky lands and near streams.

.Medical properties.-Hydrangea root has obtained a wide reputation for its action on the bladder, assisting the easy passage of gravel by relaxing the ureters, and by some supposed to help dissolve small phosphatic gravel in the kidneys. Its influence is that of a gentle relaxant with demulcent properties, like all demulcents acting on the renal passages and opening the bowels. It soothes these passages, and thus relieves the tenderness and pain caused by small calculi; and at the same time relaxes the passages somewhat, and increases the flow of urine, by which combined impressions it becomes of much service under such circumstances. It is also good in sub-acute and chronic cystitis, and similar conditions of the urethra, uterus and vagina. Much overrated by some, it has been too much neglected by others; and if used in its proper place, with due regard to its properties and. without expecting impossibilities from it, it will be found an excellent remedy. Dose of fluid extract, 10 to 20 drops.

HYDRASTIS CANADENSIS.

GOLDEN SEAL. YELLOW PUCCOON.

In his Medical Flora of 1824, Dr. C. F. Rafinesque brought this agent to professional notice as a valuable tonic. From that time it gradually grew into favor among certain classes of physicians, and has always sustained its reputation. I have employed. it liberally for more than forty years, and wrote about it freely in 1868-'69. Within the last fifteen years it has come prominently into favor; and probably has received more attention, been a subject of more investigation, enjoyed more encomiums, and come into more general use than any other vegetable remedy, except the once despised and rejected cinchona. I feel justified in here quoting portions of what I wrote and published about it in 1869 :

"This root is one of the purest tonics, the stimulating property predominating. It acts slowly and steadily. holding its influence for several hours. Its influence upon the system is very general; and there seems to be no organ or tissue but can be benefited by its appropriate use, though it is most prominently advantageous to mucous membranes, the digestive apparatus and the uterine organs. Though a stimulant, and hence sustaining to the circulation, it never excites or forces the pulse, and is unlike almost all other stimulating tonics in soothing the irritation connected with feeble and congested conditions of the mucous membranes.

"In its action on mucous membranes, hydrastis first secures the separation and discharge of any viscid secretion; then diminishes the secretion without reducing it below normal, and renders it more healthy in character, and at the same time relieves turgid conditions and achings, and disposes any ulcerated portions to heal. These actions are very decided and peculiar, and render this agent one of rare value in purulent and granular ophthalmia, ulceration of the cornea, nasal catarrh, aphthous, sore mouth, diphtheria and scarlatina, leucorrhma, catarrh of the bladder, etc. In the second stage of dysentery, chronic dysentery and diarrhea, and chronic and typhoid ulcerations of the bowels, it is unsurpassed. The ease it gives to the achings peculiar to these maladies, as also to cystic congestion and chronic difficulties of the prostrate, is gratifying."

At that time I also fully set forth its action as a stomachic tonic; its usefulness in feeble assimilation, hepatic torpor, leucorrhea, and during convalescence from acute debilitating maladies; and its advantages as an outward application in scrofulous and other low-grade ulcers, in bruises and wounds with congestion, and peculiarly in allaying the itching and preventing the pitting of small-pox. Time has fully confirmed all I said of it in this large range of usefulness.

Following my investigations of the clinical uses of the agent, in 1876 I published my conclusions that it acted as a tonic on the venous walls, reaching from the venous capillaries to the larger vessels, finally impressing the venae cavae, and thence the right side of the heart itself. It thus becomes to the venous circulation what capsicum is to the arterial circulation, though acting more slowly and more as a tonic than a stimulant. We have very few non-toxic agents that act in this manner, and probably none that equals hydrastis in reliable sustaining influence. Time has fully confirmed what I published as to the heart-tonic action of the article in 1876.

This peculiar property of hydrastis, while in no degree lessening the value of its influence upon mucous tissues, gives it a unique and must desirable place in all cases involving local or general venous feebleness, sluggishness or congestion. Probably it is by thus sustaining the portal veins that it is so beneficial in hepatic torpor and congestion, and in jaundice; and by the same action on the hemorrhoidal veins it is so useful, locally, in turgid piles. It is this property, apparently, that renders hydrastis so useful in hepatic and cardiac dropsies, and in phlegmasia dolens; while it is of secondary service, though beneficial as an adjunct to other agents, in renal dropsies.

I have tested the power of hydrastis upon the central venous system by giving it to avert and remove hepatization in pneumonia, while using suitable measures to restore the outward circulation; and the result has been greatly to my satisfaction, and in some cases so admirable as to be surprising. It is not to be set down merely as a remedy for pneumonia, for that signifies nothing as to the mode of its usefulness nor the conditions calling for its exhibition. But when given for the purpose above indicated, at the proper time, and while other medicaments are suitably directed, my experience convinces me that hydrastis is effectual in sustaining the venous pulmonary circulation and the heart, thus proving of great service against the effusion of blood in this malady. Its employment in other cases where failure of the venous centres is apparent, will suggest itself. In anaemia it thus becomes an especially desirable remedy, both by improving digestion and by sustaining the entire venous system. My practice has been to use a portion of some soluble iron salt with hydrastis, as the tartrate of iron and potassa, thus improving intestinal as well as gastric digestion.

In various local venous congestions besides portal sluggishness, hydrastis becomes serviceable. Thus, in venous hyperaemia of the kidneys, in uterine engorgement with passive haemorrhage, in menorrhagia and similar wastings, in haemorrhoids, and other like conditions, it is desirable. From its influence in diminishing uterine floodings, some have thought it possessed astringent properties; but it is effective by toning up the relaxed venous walls, thereby contracting the calibre of these vessels and thus checking the waste. It has no astringency, and hence needs, under such circumstances, to be combined with such an astringent as viburnum prunifolium, each remedy aiding the other effectively.

Locally, hydrastis is an admirable remedy in all cases that include dilatation and feebleness of the venous tissues. In every class of ulcer presenting such a condition-and what continuing ulcer does not present it-this agent can he relied on. It may be applied as a powder, in an ointment, or by poultice, as judged most advisable. Perhaps its good effects are most apparent in scrofulous sores, while internal medication is being carried on. When used on indulent sores, where the arterial capillary circulation is feeble and reparative effort is wanting, some direct stimulant should be combined with hydrastis, as ginger in mild cases and a portion of capsicum in stubborn and unimpressible cases, so long as the parts are purplish or gray. In the deep and phlegmmonous forms of erysipelas it is admirable, I am almost tempted to say indispensable, a strong infusion as a wash being soothing to the endangered nerves by sustaining the venous capillaries. Cervical ulcers and vaginal congestion are much benefited by it, in a wash or otherwise; and in chronic catarrh of the bladder it makes an admirable injection. In many cases of eczema, psoriasis and other skin diseases, it allays the irritation and tones the weakened structures; and may be mingled with glycerine and diluted.

Different alkaloids are found in hydrastis. One of these, berberine, (in commerce frequently termed hydrastia), is similar to that found in berberis vulgaris, xanthorrhiza, and some other plants.

As obtained it is in minute acicular crystals, soluble in 100 parts of cold water, less soluble in alcohol, freely soluble in hot water and hot alcohol, bitter. Berberina, as .an alkaloid, forms salts with sulphuric, phosphoric, acetic and hydro-chloric acids, commonly offered in commerce as the sulphate, phosphate and hydrochlorate of hydrastia. These are sparingly soluble, giving deep yellow and intensely bitter solutions. They are much used instead of other preparations of hydrastis, especially for washes in conjunctivitis, etc.
From one-fourth to one-half a grain to the ounce of distilled water makes a collyrium of the first value in ophthalmias and corneal ulcerations; and more than once I have seen opacity of the cornea from ulceration disappear under its use. It may be combined with alum when an astringent is needed, hut not with anything containing tannic acid. I n gastric ulcers it is excellent; also for injections to the bladder, in gonorrhoea, etc., where one to three grains may be used to the ounce. It can be combined with iron tartrate when the latter is needed, as in anaemia. Dose of hydrochlorate or sulphate, 1-15 to 1-8 of a grain.

Hydrastine is another alkaloid, obtained after the berberine has been precipitated by hydroehloric acid. It is in white or colorless crystals, nearly insoluble in water, readily soluble in alcohol and ether, tasteless. It forms salts with the acid, most of which are soluble. When hydrastine has been precipitated from water, the portiun remaining in solution is known as colorless hydrastis, and is valuable as a wash in leucorrhoea, gonorrhoea, cystic troubles, etc. It is diluted by from one to ten or more parts of water before being used; and one part of this with four to ten parts of distilled hamamelis, and borax as indicated, makes an admirable combination for these purposes.

Hydrastin is probably an impure combination of the several alkaloids. This is frequently used in those elegant preparations, parvules and granules, where fractional doses are required,-the parvules of Messrs. Warner & Co. containing 1-20 of a grain.

HYDROGEN PEROXIDE.

Water, the chemical combination of hydrogen and oxygen gases, may be made to take to itself another atom of oxygen under certain circumstances. This fact has long been known in chemistry, the resultant compound being hydrogen dioxide, or commonly called peroxide of hydrogen. It is an unstable compound, being disposed to give up its extra atom of oxygen under many trifling disturbances. The atom of oxygen thus yielded is, at the moment or liberation, nascent oxygen; and in oxidizing power is second only to ozone itself.

Hydrogen dioxide will be absorbed readily by water; and the medicinal preparation known as hydrogen peroxide is a 3 1 -5 percent solution of the chemically pure compound. This is capable of liberating fifteen times its own volume of oxygen gas, and is spoken of as a fifteen-volume solution. To preserve this from a rapid loss of its oxygen, by which it would soon he worthless, it is acidulated with 1/6000 percent of hydro-chloric acid and 1/10000 percent of phosphoric acid. As thus prepared, it constitutes the medicinal hydrogen peroxide of the shops. It is a clear liquid, slightly acid to litmus paper, parting with its second atom of oxygen and leaving only water behind if exposed to light or heated above 69° F., hence requiring to be kept in a dark and cool place.

Medical Properties.-By virtue of its readiness to liberate the extra atom of oxygen, this article becomes an active oxidizer when brought in contact with pus, degenerate tissues and decaying flesh. Advantage of this property is taken in treating abscesses, ulcers, cancers, lupus, and similar diseases when processes of suppur-ation and decay are in progress. The 15-volume solution may be used, or a 10 or 25 or 50 percent dilution of this, according to circumstances- bad cases requiring the preparation of full strength, and mild cases needing it much reduced. It is injected into suppurating cavities, using none but a glass or rubber syringe; and poured or otherwise laved upon open sores. When it comes in contact with pus the sudden liberation of oxygen causes this to bubble up into a froth; and the albumen is coagulated, and the discharge is at the same time rendered innocuous and the surface is relieved of it. Abscesses are thus improved in their contents, which can now be cleansed away easily; and sores are cleansed, decaying fibres removed, and offensive discharges removed by this peroxide, It may be used two or several times a day, as needed; and is one of the most powerful and satisfactory of antiseptic medicaments known to surgery. It is more potent than sublimate solution. which heretofore has stood at the head; and has the great advantage over that and many other antiseptics of being void of toxic properties. It accomplishes its work of purification without endangering the patient or the healthy tissues.

Besides its use for the above purposes, hydrogen peroxide is employed as a spray or wash upon suppurative and putrefactive diseases of the mucous surfaces. Thus diluted preparations, 1 to 8 or 20, are thrown into the nostrils for putrid catarrh, into the ears for catarrhal and suppurative diseases, used in the eyes for purulent and granular conjunctivitis; and some have found it valuable in gonorrhea, vaginitis, and other diseases of mucous structures. It is employed two or three times a day in these conditions, and followed by suitable medicaments. As a spray for diphtheria, and for putrid scarlatina, it is exceedingly valuable; and may be used freely every three or two hours, diluted or of full strength as needed. It may also be used as a gargle in such cases, and diluted as a mouth wash in typhoid.

I do not attempt to treat diphtheria without a steady use of hydrogen peroxide, accompanied with other suitable agents. It arrests putrefaction, softens the exudate and hastens its removal, and averts the dangers of septic absorption; and this without any regard to the microbe theory, as it probably destroys the microbes while doing its other work.

ICHTYOL-ICHTHYOL.

By distillation from a bituminous substance found in a district of the Tyrol is obtained a nearly black mass of the consistency of vaseline or of a very thick oil. It has a strong and disagreeable odor, mixes readily with vaseline, glycerine and the fixed oils, is partly soluble in both alcohol and ether, but dissolves readily in a mixture of the two menstrua, and may be made into an emulsion with water. The bituminous substance is rich in the fossilized remains of fishes; and the ichtyol obtained by dry distillation contains considerable quantities of sulphur and phosphorus with fishy oils.

Medical Uses.--Ichtyol at present enjoys prominence as an outward application in psoriasis and humid eczema. An ointment is said to allay the intense itching speedily, and soon to dry up eczematous discharges, abate the pain and effect a cure. In dry eczema it promptly quiets the pain and pruritus. A solution in equal parts of ether and alcohol may be used for the same purpose either as a wash or a spray, generally followed by an ointment of the article. It is also used in other painful and burning skin diseases, as acne, prurigo, favus, etc. In parasitic diseases, as ringworm, it is reputed rapidly effective. Some speak highly of it in pruritus vulvae and ani, a weak ointment being used; and strong ointments are given warm praise in chronic rheumatism. In short, as in the case of most new agencies, it has been made a "fad" and used for almost everything with such loud encomiums as would throwaway all other outward medicaments; hy which extravagance the real place it should occupy is covered with confusion.

Ichtyol has been used inwardly, chiefly in catarrh of the larynx and trachea with hypersecretion. For these purposes it is employed by adding a small portion to hot water and inhaling the fumes. In gonorrhea, syphilis and scrofula it has been given in doses of 3 to 5 drops, by capsule or pill, three times a day. Also as an emulsion by injection to the urethra and vagina in gonorrhea and leucorrhea. The offensive odor of the article stands in the way of its use, especially of its internal administration. Much of this odor is covered by the addition of a little vanilin. From its outward application a miliary eruption may arise; which it is said may be prevented by mingling it with equal parts of sweet oil and lime water, and avoiding cotton or other warm dressing. Ointments may be made of varying strength, from 5 to 50 percent in lard or vaseline, that of 20 percent being the average for moist eczema; yet it needs watching.

INGLUVIN.

Our grandmothers were accustomed to boiling the gizzards of chickens and giving the broth to arrest vomiting and to strengthen weak stomachs. It was a homely but an efficient procedure; and what was once laughed at as the "whim of old women," has been utilized by science as a valuable truth.

Ingluvin is prepared from the gizzard of chickens, as pepsin is obtained from the stomach of hogs and pancreatin from the sweet-breads of cattle. It is a greenish-gray powder, of slightly bitter taste, insoluble in water. As an aid to gastric digestion it is mild, not supplying a lack of gastric juice so much as soothing the nerves of the stomach and imparting tone to the peptic glands. Its best action is shown when a weak stomach becomes irritable and food is vomited. Such cases occur in the reflex vomiting of pregnancy, and also of hysteria, in both of which conditions ingluvin generally proves quite effective. Infantile vomiting is usually much benefited by it; and the article deserves much confidence in all these classes of troublesome stomach weakness. Dose two to five grains at the time of meals, or soon after. It may be given in milk.

INULA HELENIUM.

ELECAMPANE.

Both in family and professional practice the root of elecampane has long been a favorite stimulating expectorant and emmenagogue. Helenin has recently been prepared from it, a white crystalline body analogous to the concrete oils, of an aromatic odor and bitter taste, soluble in alcohol and ether, insoluble in water.

Helenin is a concentrated agent, sharply stimulating, acting on the pulmonary membranes and circulation. It is used in depressed conditions, as bronchorrhea, threatening gangrene, etc. Antiseptic powers have been attributed to it, as it overcomes the fetor of certain expectorations; but I judge it is beneficial rather by stimulating the pulmonary capillaries than by any power to arrest decay of tissue. It has been supposed capable of destroying tubercle bacilli, but it is simply a sharp stimulating expectorant. Dose, one-eighth to one-half of a grain every three or two hours. Large doses may excite emesis. Best given in capsule with glycrrhiza. Too potent for children.

LIGUSTICUM FILICINUM.

OSHA ROOT, COLORADO LOVAGE.

Among the popular medicinal plants furnished by the Rocky Mountains is the Osha root. It is common through New Mexico, Colorado, Utah and Wyoming; thriving on damp grounds at an elevation of from 8,000 to 10,000 feet. Dr. Watson places it as Ligusticum filicinum; and it seems to be a variety of, or the same as, L. scopularum of Gray. It is a lovage, allied to the Angelicre; in the family of Umbelliferre which furnishes the edible parsnip and carrot, the medicinal fennel, dill, anise, caraway, celery, coriander and parsley; and the poisonous conium and cicuta.

Among the people of the above section. osha root is greatly prized as a remedy for coughs, and is an ingredient of several proprietary medicines. Like so many other plants of the same family, its seeds contain a number of oil-tubes that yield a volatile oil that is aromatic and pungent; and the roots, which have a strong odor and taste similar to angelica, contain both an aromatic and a fixed oil, and a considerable amount of resin.

Medical Properties.-Osha root is a stimulating aromatic with some relaxing properties, rather pungent in taste, acting promptly. It expends the greater portion of its influence on the respiratory passages; a small portion on the genito-urinary apparatus, and at the same time is warming to the stomach and carminative. From the relaxing property it contains, it is a good antispasmodic; and its sustaining influence on the capillaries of the mucosa leaves a somewhat tonic impression. It is used mostly in coughs, proving expectorant and antispasmodic in a desirable degree, allaying tickling in the throat, averting paroxysms of coughing, and overcoming capillary congestion in bronchitis and catarrh. In this particular field of action it will be found a most desirable remedy, and may be associated with prunus. glycrrhiza and similar agents. The people chew small pieces, swallowing the abundant salivary secretion it excites. In fine powder it is used as a catarrh snuff. A warm infusion promotes perspiration, and also acts well in restoring recently obstructed menstruation. It has a certain amount of emmenagogue tonic action, and can no doubt be utilized as an aromatic adjuvant to uterine tonics. It is best made into a syrup, or into a lozenge containing a definite amount of the resin. Colorado druggists handle the article locally; but it well deserves being brought upon the general market, preferable to many foreign remedies.

Ligusticum levesticum, or European lovage, is an allied plant of southern Europe, the root, stem, and seeds of which have long been in use by the people. It has a stronger aroma, a more pungent taste and larger amounts of resin than our L. filicinum. As a diffusively stimulating and antispasmodic article, its chief use has been by warm infusion, or tincture given in warm water, as a carminative and emmenagogue, in flatulent colic, suppressed menses from cold, etc. It is seldom used by the profession, except as a desirable adjuvant to bitter and more permanent remedies.

LIPPIA MEXICANA.

LIPPIA.

Mexico, the West Indies and southward furnish us this trailing, shrubby evergreen of the verbena family. Its leaves contain a volatile oil of pleasant odor and sweetish taste.

Medical Properties.-The leaves and stems of lippia are distinctly stimulating, with a full share of relaxing properties and some demulcent. Their action is quite diffusive, and hence transient. Given in considerable doses of powder, their effects are mostly limited to the stomach, and cause nausea despite their pleasant taste. In concentrated tincture they promptly increase expectoration, allay tickling of the throat, and arrest spasmodic coughs. Large doses will flush the face and favor perspiration.

The article is chiefly valuable for its action on the larynx and bronchi, being a desirable antispasmodic expectorant in colds, coughs, laryngeal and bronchial catarrhs. It is too transient to be of much service when used alone, but is a fine adjunct to more permanent agents, as prunus, aralia, liriodendron, etc. A highly concentrated tincture is better than a fluid extract, and more miscible with syrups. Dose of such tincture, 2 to 10 drops, as needed.

LITHIUM COMPOUNDS.

As a solvent of uric acid deposits, the compounds of lithium have long been known, yet used but sparingly by the profession. Recent prominence has been given to them by the extensive advertising of lithia waters, which has drawn toward them the attention of physicians and people. In this instance the energy of commercial enterprise has been a pronounced benefit to the profession, which cannot he said in favor of all enterprise.

The alkali, LITHIA, is not abundant; and its chief source is in several mineral waters. in which it is found in quite small quantities, usually in the form of a soluble carbonate or bicarbonate. Its great advantage over other alkalies and alkaline carbonates lies in its quality of forming compounds with uric acid that are soluble. Other alkalies enter into combination with that acid and form salts, but these salts are insoluble; whereas the lithia and uric acid salts are very soluble, and thus furnish a ready form for the removal of uric acid from the system. The equivalent or combining power of alkali lithia with uric acid is also very great; hence a small quality of lithia is sufficient to effect a large purpose in the animal economy.

Uric acid, in some form, is present in the system in three painful and serious classes of maladies,-Gravel, Rheumatism, and Gout. It is in these, and for its solvent effects, that Lithia is employed. That it enters the blood is abundantly shown by analysis; and while chemical therapy is far from commendable in some instances, there is no reasonable ground to question the benefits of lithia in these connections. It cannot establish the functions, nor equalize the circulation, nor sustain the nervous system and the digestion, as are necessary in the three classes of maladies named; but it manifestly reaches and dissolves the uric add accumulations so detrimental in them all, and presents them in that soluble form which the kidneys can eliminate. That lithia compounds will do this, and aid other suitable measures in giving effective relief in those maladies, is not a question of hope, but has been proven abundantly. And in correcting the uric acid diathesis, it benefits this form of asthma.

Lithia is used largely by way of the different spring waters containing it, of which several are on the market and all of about the same qualities. It may also be used in the form of either the carbonate or citrate, given in water or added to any suitable pharmacal preparation.

LITHIUM CARBONATE is a white, odorless powder, of distinct alkaline reaction, soluble in about 130 parts of cold or boiling water, permanent in the air, insoluble in alcohol. Its combining number is very low, hence its neutralizing power is very great. It increases the flow of urine, prevents the formation of insoluble salts of uric acid, and acts as a solvent on such salts when they have been deposited about the joints in rheumatism, or in the kidneys or bladder. Dose 5 to 10 grains three times a day in water or in carbonic acid water. A weak solution of it has been injected into the bladder to disintegrate calculi.

LITHIUM CITRATE is prepared from carbonate of lithium with citric acid, mixing the two in solution till effervescence ceases, then evaporating and drying carefully. It is a white powder, without odor faintly alkaline to the taste, but neutral in reaction, slowly deliquescent in the air and hence should be kept closely stoppered. It has an advantage over the carbonate in being much more soluble, one part dissolving in less than six parts of cold water and in two and one-half parts of boiling water; slightly soluble in alcohol. Its taste is much more pleasant than that of the carbonate, and it is not so likely to irritate the stomach. It is used for the same purposes as the carbonate, in doses of from 10 to 20 grains.

Effervescing tablets of lithium carbonate are put on the market and are a very pleasant form for its administration, one tablet dissolved in a glass of water being a dose. It may be drank during effervescence, or after this has subsided. To avoid surcharging the blood with lithium, it is advisable not to continue the use of any of its preparations longer than one month, and then allow an intermission of one or two weeks.

LYCOPUS VIRGINICUS.
BUGLE WEED.

Bugle weed is common throughout the United States, growing in moist and shady situations. An erect herb, seldom branched, 12 to 18 inches high; leaves opposite, sessile, broad lanceolate, rough, purplish, with glandular dots beneath; flowers very small, white, in small axillary whorls.

Medical Properties.-I previously wrote of the good qualities of the entire herb bugle weed, as a soothing astringent of mild power, and excellent in pulmonary and other hemorrhages. Further experience has shown that it has a desirable influence upon the venous circulation, even reaching to the right side of the heart and sustaining it.

This power is mild, and is distinctly connected with a calmative nervine property; and the effect of the remedy is quieting but in no sense narcotic on the heart, and at the same time tonic. It thus serves a good purpose in numerous cases where there is cardiac excitement with nervous irritability, lessening the frequency of the pulse and giving it more firmness. Used outwardly and given inwardly, it improves the tone of the vein walls in weakness and varices; and is a serviceable article in hemorrhages, haematuria and chyluria.

LYCOPUS EUROPAEUS, or bitter bugle, has a sharply angled stem; leaves narrow, 2 to 4 inches long, on petioles, frequently lobed. It is much more bitter than the former, and acts largely on the glandular structures as an alterative, and has been used successfully in malaria. These plants well deserve much more attention than they have received.

MAGNESIUM MILK.

Under the title Milk of Magnesium, a liquid preparation of magnesium oxide is put upon the market. Bottled at the moment of chemical interchange, it remains a milky fluid until exposure to the air slowly converts it into the magnesium carbonate. It is a mild alkaline preparation, much more acceptable to the stomach than the powdered carbonates, and also much more easily administered. It is used in any case where acidity of the stomach and intestines calls for a mild alkali, in diarrhea and similar bowel troubles, sour eructations, etc. It has over potassium and sodium bicarbonates the advantages of pleasantness and mildness; and is one of the more desirable agents of its class.

MALT.

Malt is the result of causing barley to germinate under moisture and a certain regulated degree of heat, then drying it upon the floor, and afterwards kiln-drying it at a temperature that will effectually kill the young plant germ without scorching the mass. In this process, and as a first result in the process, there is developed in the grain a small quantity of a peculiar principle called diastase. Barley contains only about two parts of diastase in a thousand of the grain; oats and wheat produce a yet smaller percentage of it.

When the diastase has been developed in the earlier steps of the germinating process, it acts upon the starchy elements of the grain and converts these into soluble forms of dextrine and maltose sugar. Diastase has a peculiar power in thus preparing amylaceous substances for uses in the body; and the ptyalin of saliva and the enzyme of the pancreas and Brunner's glands are properly animal diastase; and its presence effects the digestion of starchy foods, while its deficiency or absence leaves this class of foods more or less undigested and gives rise to one form of dyspepsia.

In therapeutics, malt is used for the purpose of obtaining from it the nutritive soluble principles of dextrin and maltose into which its starch has been converted by the above-named action of the diastase. For this purpose, a decoction of malt may be made by boiling two or three ounces of barley in a quart of water for half an hour, and straining. This decoction is demulcent and nutritious, and its use at meals or soon after will materially aid the process of starch digestion. An extract of malt is made by macerating the coarse powder of malt with water for several hours, at a temperature of about 125° to 130° F.; then straining with strong pressure and carefully evaporating the liquid to the consistence of honey.

This is the true extract of malt; and a good article should contain no free starch, nor should the manufacturer adulterate it with glucose. It is an excellent nutrient and promoter of starch digestion, very serviceable for children, feeble women and convalescents generally.

When a decoction of malt is allowed to proceed to a certain stage of fermentation, and hops are added, it forms what is termed wort, and from this is made the various malt drinks of ale, beer and lager beer. Too many of the liquid malt preparations put upon the market under the name of Malt, and Extract of Malt, are nothing more than individual manufactures of beer, and often with considerable amounts of glucose added to give them" body" and render the taste of hops less noticeable.

MANGANESE.

It has been claimed that manganese is a powerful oxygenized of the blood, enriching it in red corpuscles more rapidly and extensively than can be done by any of the preparations of iron. This claim is based upon the fact that minute quantities of manganese exist in the blood; and that this metal is a powerful medium for conveying oxygen from one body to another in the chemist's laboratory, and therefore should he expected to do the same in the animal economy. As the human system and its functions are things quite different from the chemist's crucibles and pipes and reagents, and cannot be built up and set in motion in his laboratory, the chemical claim for the action of manganese is deceptive. It must be judged by the clinical results of its use. These seem to be analogous to those of the non-toxic preparations of iron, and apparently are more potent than the iron compounds. Manganese and iron are sometimes associated in a dialyzed solution; and manganese and peptones are also offered. So far as my experience has gone, it is quite favorable to the latter combination for improving gastric and intestinal digestion and appetite in pale and feeble subjects, especially children. Albuminate, peptonate and saccharate of manganese are soluble in water, forming a brown solution of a slightly astringent yet pleasant taste, and are used in the same way as iron albuminate and haemogallol.

MENTHOL.

Menthol is a white, crystalline, camphoraceous body deposited from oil of peppermint under the influence of a very low degree of cold (-10°F.) The peppermint oil of China and Japan furnishes the supply, as the European and American peppermint plant does not yield an oil sufficiently rich in menthol. The crystals are in cylinders packed together, resembling epsom salts, and of very light weight. A powerful peppermint odor comes from it, though less pungent than the oil; its taste is sharp and penetrates the whole mouth, causing the peppermint-like sense of coolness afterwards. It dissolves readily in alcohol, is but slightly soluble in water, dissolves in fixed and in volatile oils, and volatilizes when heated. Like camphor, it will slowly evaporate and disappear if left exposed at ordinary temperatures.

Medical Properties.-In Japan and China, menthol camphor has long been used for neuralgic headache. A stick or pencil of it rubbed lightly on the forehead causes a feeling of coldness and gives quick relief to the suffering. Passed along the sciatic nerve it relieves sciatica; and a few grains in a carious tooth stops toothache, or it may be dissolved in spirits and applied. Its mode o{action is not well understood, but its effects are almost instantaneous, and it may also be said of them that they are not permanent in all cases. Antiseptic properties are attributed to it; and so it has been lauded as an inhalent, through neat menthol tubes, in catarrh, diphtheria, etc. As a stimulating inhalent it is good, either using the crystals or a solution. For other uses it may be dissolved in oil, vaseline or albolene; and 10 grains or less to the ounce of albolene may be used as a throat spray and to reach the Eustachian tube. For some years it was a "fad," and put to extraordinary uses, as in piles, phthisis, asthma, etc.

OENOTHERA BIENNIS.

EVENING PRIMROSE, SCARISH, SUNDROP, CURE-ALL.

A handsome plant, found throughout the United States, its large and bright yellow flowers opening in the evening.

Medical Properties.-Scabish leaves are of mild power, combining-some stimulation with considerable relaxation; acting on the peripheries of sensory nerves, relieving local and reflex excitability. A large portion of its action is directed to the pneumogastric nerve, making it of service in asthma with gastric irritability.

It has proven useful in hyper-sensitiveness of the stomach with indigestion, uterine irritability, hysteria, hysterical vomiting, tenesmus, spasmodic cough, and other difficulties of reflex origin. Some have used it in facial neuralgia and in angina pectoris; but I think it is not adapted to the conditions in such cases, where more distinct stimulation is needed.

From its soothing, quieting influence on excited nerve peripheries, it has been spoken of as a sedative; and this term usually conveys the idea of narcosis. My experience with it has given me no occasion to associate it with any degree of narcosis; but to class it as a relaxing nervine leaving a slightly tonic impression. It is a good application to irritable ulcers. Dose of the fluid extract, half a drachm or more every three or four hours, or smaller doses at shorter intervals.

ORTHOSIPHON STAMINEUS.

JAVA TEA.

As yet the American use of this plant is but limited, but its use in the East Indies and continental Europe has become considerable. It is a member of the family of labiatre, native to Java, Hindostan and Australia. The leaves are aromatic, diffusively stimulant and somewhat astringent. Their action is directed chiefly to the kidneys and bladder, increasing the flow of urine and facilitating the expulsion of gravel. Also of value in relieving the distress of renal colic, chronic cystitis, etc.

In ascites due to cirrhosis it has reduced the abdomen, and caused the urine to become abundant and clear. An infusion may be used freely; or the fluid extract in doses of 10 to 20 drops, in water, three or foul' times a day.

OXYDENDRUM ARBOREUM.

SOUR WOOD, SORREL TREE, ELK WOOD.

This member of the family of heaths is a tree common in the valleys of the Alleghanies, through Ohio, Pennsylvania, Virginia and southward. Attains a height of 20 to 50 feet, with tough, smooth, narrow and pointed leaves 4 to 6 inches long, resembling the peach. The botanical family to which it belongs abounds in medicinal plants, including uva ursi, epigea, gaultheria, vaccinium and others.

Medical Properties.-The leaves of this tree contain a free acid, and are distinctly and pleasantly sour to the taste. They have long had a popular use as a grateful drink in fevers, satisfying thirst and increasing the flow of urine. Both the leaves and bark have come into use as strong diuretics with some tonic properties, and have gained some celebrity in anasarca, hydrops pericardii, and other dropsies. Reports of their effects in such conditions are encouraging; although temporary relief by merely rapid drainage through the kidneys is far from being a cure of dropsy, As an adjunct to other and more permanently tonic agents it deserves attention. A solid extract may be made into pills, and from 6 to 10 given in twenty-four hours. Dose of fluid extract, half a drachm to a drachm every six or four hours.

PANCREATINE.

For a number of years the pancreatic juice of the hog has been upon the market in the form, usually, of a saccharated powder. It is obtained by macerating the cut-up pancreas in water acidulated with hydrochloric acid, filtering and adding a strong solution of sodium chloride. The pancreatine rises to the top, and is gathered, washed, dried without heat, and then rubbed up with sugar of milk.

Pancreatine is used to aid intestinal digestion by there forming an emulsion with the fats in the food, which is the physiological work of the pancreatic secretion. In a smaller measure it promotes the digestion of starchy elements. When these processes in digestion fail, pancreatine is serviceable to assist them. Consumptives, those with tabes, and very lean people, can use this article to advantage. It has no influence on gastric digestion, which is aided by pepsin; and because of its inability in this respect, it has by many been set aside. Use it in its proper connection and it will be found valuable. It is commonly advised to be taken with the meals; but this brings it in contact with the fullest flow of gastric juice, by which it is practically nullified. It needs to be associated with an alkali, such as soda bicarbonate; and my own practice has been to give 5 grains pancreatine with 8 or 10 grains of the soda, an hour to an hour and a half after the meals. It is insoluble in water, but may be exhibited in water or milk.

Milk gently heated with pancreatine and soda bicarbonate is soon changed in its characters by the emulsifying or "predigestion" of its fats. Such milk is said to be "pancreatized," and is then much more easy of digestion by children and invalids. If the process is too much prolonged, the taste becomes unpleasant. When prepared, a "day's supply should be kept in a cold place, and given alone or mingled with other foods as desired. It is a good food product for summer complaints, marasmic children, and whenever digestion of milk-fats is ill-performed.

PARACOTO.

From central Brazil and Bolivia come two barks, known as coto and paracoto. At first they were supposed to be one and the same, but latterly they have been spoken of as two barks of the same class, though the tree from which they are obtained has not been determined. It is obtained through the missions of Bolivia, and is thought to be a species (or two species) of Nectandria. This is a very indeterminate manner of adjusting an agent; but the article to which the Bolivian name paracoto is applied is of such potency, and apparently so peculiar in its action, that it deserves more careful investigation.

Medical Properties.-Paracoto is a sharp aromatic, slightly bitter, and in large doses biting, exciting eructations. By the people it is used for rheumatism and toothache; its chief use by the profession is in the treatment of diarrhrea. Its use here seems to secure admirable results; and this not by any astringent action whatever, but apparently from its sustaining action on the intestinal circulation and nerves, whereby it promotes intestinal digestion. It seems also to have a measure of power to delay intestinal fermentative changes.

The reports of its beneficial influence in ordinary diarrhoea from indigestion are numerous; also in intestinal catarrh, the diarrhoea of phthisis and tubercular night-sweats. The fluid extract is given in doses of 5 to 10 drops, usually in mucilage with some light aromatic. Large doses irritate and may excite vomiting.

PASSIFLORA INCARNATA.

PASSION FLOWER.

This American plant has come into prominence recently. It is placed among the nervines, and glowing accounts of its power to induce sleep have been given. From this use narcotic properties were attributed to it. From my own experience, and from that of several professional friends, it is my belief that the agent is not a narcotic in any sense.

Passiflora seems to be a genial relaxant to the sensory nervous system, with a small measure of mild nervine-tonic power. It quite resembles that most valuable of non-toxic nervines, cypripedium, but it chiefly influences the spinal sensory system rather than the peripheries. This makes it peculiarly soothing in all nervous irritations, as neuralgia, insomnia, chorea, infantile convulsions, spinal sensitiveness, hysteria and general restlessness. Its action is prompt and pleasant; the sense of relief it gives is agreeable, and I have not seen it accompanied or followed by any symptoms that intimated physiological disturbance. Dose of fluid extract, 10 to 20 drops every three or two hours.

PAULLINIA SORBILIS.

GUARANA.

A climbing shrub of BraziL with large pinnate leaves and bearing a grape-like fruit, having a seed not unlike a small hazel-nut. The seeds are used in medicine, being washed, dried, roasted like coffee, made into small rolls with a little water, and then slowly dried again. In this form it comes to market. It contains a bitter alkaloidal principle called guaranine, which resembles caffeine. The natives of the Amazon regions use it for a beverage, as we use coffee and tea.

Medical Properties.-Guarana was introduced as a remedy for sick headache; but that gives no indication of the action of the agent. I have employed it in migraine and several other maladies, and have not always been pleased with its influence on the system. It increases the cerebral circulation, causing the face to flush, brain to feel full, and the mind to be first excited and afterwards drowsy. Such physiological influences suggest stimulation of the cerebral center with increased blood pressure, followed by dilatation of the veins and sinuses and slowing of the flow. I have seen the flush followed by pallor, a sense of oppression at the heart, excitement and then reduction of the general circulation, and slow respiration with sighing.

Such a line of symptoms has made me doubtful of its being sanative, especially as those who are most accustomed to use it say that "in overdoses it is poisonous."

Its influence in sick headache is promptly stimulating toward the brain; and as that influence is frequently needed in the condition of cerebral anaemia present in some attacks of this malady, guarana gives much relief in such cases, but is of no use in cases having a gastric or an hepatic origin, and where the face is already flushed with dilated vessels. It has been given in painful diarrhooa, colic and neuralgia. Some have employed it as an antispasmodic in asthma.

Observation has not satisfied me as to its mode of bringing benefit, and it too often seems to leave behind a sense of oppression and undefinable malaise that is not to be desired. I give it a place out of respect to many friends who think well of it; and will be glad if their experience and that of others shall prove more favorable to it than my own has done.

PELLETIERINE.
PUNICINE.

Pomegranate root has long been used for the expulsion of tapeworm, and with gratifying success; but the article deteriorates by age, and often is inert from this cause. Pelletier, of France, succeeded in obtaining from it an alkaloid liquid in its commercial form, soluble in water, and somewhat volatile. This is called Pelletierine; and is reported to be a very efficient taeniacide. The sulphate of pelletierine is the salt oftenest used; and, as this is likely to be absorbed by the stomach before reaching the worm in the bowel, a little tannic acid is often added to it to delay it. The tannate is preferable, and is a tasteless powder.

Moving the bowels by a laxative or enema in the afternoon, the patient uses milk for supper, takes a drink of water and no food in the morning, and five minutes after the pelletierine, and in fifteen or twenty minutes a quick physic, as senna infusion or oil. The article causes dizziness for a time, but the entire worm is likely to be passed soon. Dose of the tannate for an adult, 20 grains; for delicate women and youths of about I5 years, 12 grains; for children of 10 to 12 years, 2 to 8 grains.

PEPSINUM-PEPSIN.

Pepsin is the digestive principle obtained from the peptic glands of the stomach of the sheep or hog. For a number of years, it appeared upon the market as a saccharated powder, the admixture of sugar of milk seeming to be necessary to furnish a permanent product by the methods formerly followed. This gave room for much deception. Better methods of manufacture now prevail; and pepsin commonly appears in scales, known as "scale pepsin."

The chief value of the article lies in its solvent power upon albumen. The strength of the agent is tested by this action upon the coagulated white of egg, a fairly good pepsin being able to dissolve 1,000 or more times its own hulk. Of late, this strength has been quite exceeded by several manufacturers. Some scale pepsins retain an unpleasant odor, which is not to their credit.

Pepsin is a distinct aid to gastric digestion, to be used when the gastric juice is deficient and the stomach is weak. It acts chiefly upon albuminous foods, in a small degree upon fibrin and casein. It does not act upon starches, sugars or fats; and hence is of no service for intestinal indigestion. It acts in the presence of acids; but is rendered inactive by the presence of alkalies. Hence pepsin is usually given in company with some acid which renders it soluble in water. Hydrochloric acid has commonly been used to acidulate the water in which the pepsin was to be given. A much better solvent is found in lactic acid, five drops for ten grains in a table-spoon or more of water. It is dissolved and well preserved by glycerine diluted. The powder called lactopeptine is thus prepared on sugar of milk, and is a fine article of this class. A small quantity of citric acid, or a little good cider vinegar. may be used for the same purpose. Alcohol damages pepsin, and "wines" of pepsin are of inferior power. Dose for an adult, 5 to 10 grains of scale pepsin just before or immediately after meals.

PEPTENZYME.

The article offered under this name claims to be a combination containing the digestive ferments produced in the seven classes of glands concerned in digestive processes, namely: the salivary, peptic, pancreatic. hepatic, splenic, Brunner's and Lieberkuhn's glands.

Each of these glands has a work of its own in preparing foods for the uses of the body; and their combined action is necessary to a satisfactory completion of the digestive function.

It is on this basis that peptenzyme has been prepared, aiming in the one article to combine the digestive ferments of the different glands in proper proportions. The high character of the house presenting the article is guarantee of integrity; it then remains to test the article on its merits. Competent gentlemen have experimented with it carefully, to determine whether the presence of one ferment would interfere with the action of another; it naturally suggesting itself that such would be the fact. So far as such experiments have gone, no such interference has been observed, but rather they tend to prove that one prepares the way for the better action of the other, throughout the series in association. That would be a fine advantage in the use of such an article, seeing that it does not stop with aiding gastric digestion; which is completed in from two to three hours, but continues giving help through the entire period occupied by intestinal digestion, which is not usually finished till twelve or more hours after a meal has been eaten.

My experience with this agent has been very satisfactory. It promotes appetite and increases nutrition, acting favorably in atonic dyspepsia, starchy indigestion, vomiting of food, derangement of the stomach during pregnancy, etc. I believe the profession will be advantaged by becoming familiar with it. Prepared in powder, tablets, and as an elixir. The elixir may be combined with euonymus, hydrastis, cascura, or other suitable agent as required. Given just before meals.

PEUMUS BOLDUS.
BOLDO.

An evergreen tree from the hillsides of Chili, where its fruit is eaten. Also called Boldo fragrans, under which name it has been employed in Chili, France and Germany for twenty years.

The leaves are fragrant, containing a quantity of an essential oil; and a glucoside principle, boldine, is obtained from the leaves and stems.

Medical Properties.-Boldo is an aromatic diffusive stimulant, with balsamic and fair tonic properties in connection with a mucilage. It acts largely upon mucous structures, including those of the kidneys, bladder and gall ducts; and is adapted to depressed conditions. It is of distinct service in the latter stages of blenorrhagia, chronic catarrh of the bladder, biliary catarrh with occlusion of the ducts, as a stomachic with bitter tonics for atonic dyspepsia, and for dislodging worms by disturbing their mucous nests. Without increasing the general circulation, it improves the smaller local circulation of the stomach and intestines, and becomes a suitable remedy in convalescence from adynamic fevers and other low conditions. Chapoteau and some other observers have found it distinctly increases the elimination of urea. For chronic hepatic troubles its powers have been somewhat overdrawn; but it is of service if we bear in mind that it opens a free passage for bile by aiding the expulsion of mucus from the ducts. Best used as an adjunct to other medicines, the fluid extract, which is not miscible with water, being given in doses of 1 to 3 or more drops.

PHYTOLACCA DECANDRA.
POKE, SCOKE, GARGET.

Of late years this common plant has come into notice anew, the former opinions in its favor having proven unwarranted and the use of its root having been almost or entirely discontinued on account of its dangerous action. Latterly it has been lauded again for rheumatic difficulties, as an agent to abort mammary abscesses. in granular conjunctivitis, and as a general alterative in cutaneous diseases. I have watched the agent carefully, and am not at all prepared to accept the ardent reports of its merits, but instead to place this root as a harsh, irritating and quite undesirable article. Its first impression is that of a slow and nauseating relaxant, followed by an irritating impression on the stomach and bowels. In any considerable quantity it induces slow emesis, with a most uncomfortable, persistent and distressing sense of prostration. Moderate doses are purgative, at times proving drastic and weakening. More than once I have been called to treat a very intractable form of intestinal irritation manifestly brought about by small doses of the fluid extract of poke root, the tenderness and weakness of the bowels persisting for weeks and being disposed to return after an interval of months. A number of physicians report weakness, drowsiness, dizziness and disturbed vision following its use, and in several well-attested instances it has extended a sad irritation to the spinal cord.

Such facts do not encourage the placing of this article among sanative agents, and verify the popular opinion that it is a severe and truly poison-ous agent.

Phytolacca berries have at times been suspected of having narcotic properties; but I have used them extensively for many years, and have never seen any narcotic or other undesirable action from them. They are an almost pure relaxant, slowly influencing the glandular system and serous tissues, and are admirable in sub-acute and chronic rheumatism, scrofula, and most cutaneous diseases. Because of their excess of relaxation they should be combined with stimulants and tonics, as stillingia, corydalis, xanthoxylum, etc.

A so-called "active principle" of these berries has been put upon the market as a proprietary medicine under the name of phytolline, as an agent to reduce excessive obesity. This idea is drawn from the fact in natural history that birds eating these berries become thin. I do not know how reliable the article may be in this respect.

PICRAMNIA.

CASCARA AMARGA, HONDURAS BARK.

From the similarity of the common names, this article is often taken to be similar to cascara sagrada. Such is not the case; for this agent belongs to some indeterminate species of Picramnia (or Picrrena) and is allied to the quassia family, whereas cascara sagrada is one of the buckthorns.

Medical Properties.-As a stimulating alterative of the tonic class, the bark of this shrub enjoys a high reputation among the people of Mexico and southward. Noting this popular estimate, it has been introduced to the profession; and reports from many physicians show it to be an article of potent qualities. Its chief use has been in the treatment of secondary and tertiary syphilis; and it seems slowly but effectually to eliminate that poison from the system through the skin and kidneys; also building up digestion. It increases the amount of solids from the kidneys, which gives it a place in certain chronic nephritic torpors. It also establishes a tonic condition through the mucous membranes, and has been of service in some severe cases of ozoena. That it establishes the cutaneous function thoroughly, is evident from the results of its use in dry and chaffy skin and the scaly diseases of syphilis. An alkaloidal principle seems to exist in it.

Evidently the article deserves investigation, for the reports already received are explicitly in its favor, and my own experience confirms them. Its action is slow and permanent. Dose of the fluid extract, 10 to 30 drops three times a day; of the powdered extract, 5 to 10 grains.

POLYMNIA UVEDALIA.

BEARSFOOT, LEAF CUP.

A coarse looking member of the composite family, found in moist places from New York westward and southward. Its strong and pubescent stem rises 3 to 8 feet; lower leaves a foot or so more in length and nearly as broad.

Medical Properties.-The root is a stimulant and relaxant, seeming to exert an influence on the secernent structures, and acting rather vigorously. It has been used outwardly to promote the absorption of glandular thickenings and deposits, and as a counter-stimulant over local inflammations. Among the conditions to which these actions adapt it are enlarged spleen and caked breast; and its efficacy in both these cases places it among our unique and potent agencies. It has been employed over an enlarged and painful liver, congested ovaries, scrofulous swellings, rheumatic thickenings, pleuritic sufferings, etc. From the relief it usually gives, it has sometimes been spoken of as an anodyne; but there is no narcotic property in it, and it abates suffering apparently by relaxing the serous and fibrous tissues while stimulating the absorption of deposits and preventing capillary stasis with its attendant dangers.

Outwardly employed as an ointment of four ounces of fluid extract in half a pound of lard, heated 30 minutes, and the liquid poured off when nearly cold. This is rubbed over the part twice a day. Inwardly 2 to 5 drops of the fluid extract are given three times a day; but it is not often used inwardly.

POLYSOLVE.

SOLVINE, SODIUM SULPHO-RICINATE.

When a triglyceride of a fatty acid, or when any of the fatty acids themselves (as the oleic), is treated with concentrated sulphuric acid, the resultant compound is sulphoricinic acid. Neutralizing this with sodium hydrate furnishes sodium sulphoricinate, commonly known as Polysolve.

It is a somewhat syrupy liquid of brownish color, readily soluble or miscible with water or alcohol. As yet, its principal use has been as a solvent to other drugs, such as sulphur, iodine, etc. A considerable number: of such agents are acted on by it. Its own action is mild and agreeable; and it seems probable that much use may be made of it for external purposes. A solution of sulphur in polysolve has been spoken of under sulphur.

PROTONUCLEIN.

This is offered to the profession as a product of blood nuclein, “derived from the lymphoid structures of healthy animals, without the use of any chemical." It is therefore classed as a physiological agent, the especial influence of which is to excite the leucocytes or white corpuscles to increased action, and to furnish them with material from which to construct proteids. On the leucocytes and their vigor depends the power of the system to resist toxic influences; hence the claims for protonuclein are that it destroys toxic germs by a physiological action and assists in building up the system from debility and waste. Its internal use is commended in anaemia, neurasthenia, diphtheria, la grippe, general sepsis, and all diseases of prostration. Locally it is advised on every degenerate grade of ulcers, including the diphtheritic sores, lupus and cancer; in all of which it is said to arouse a healthy and curative action. Not having used the article to an extent that would justify a personal opinion, this outline of its character and uses is based upon general reports from the profession. So far as noticed, all report warmly in its favor; and the article seems to be a desirable one from the physiological standpoint.

Used inwardly in tablet or powder, 3 to 5 or more grains an hour before meals. For outward application, it is prepared in a form of powder termed Special, the powder for internal use not being of use on ulcers.

RAPHIDOPHORA VITIENSIS.

TONGA.

Fiji Island natives are said to have used for centuries an article which they call tonga. It comes to market in different forms of leaf, fibre and bark, and is supposed to be obtained from the Raphidophora vitiensis. A reputation is associated with it as an agent for simple and uncomplicated neuralgia, where the suffering is not associated with inflammation. So far as I have observed the reports it seems to act by soothing the nerve peripheries and not by narcotic influence. If this proves to be the fact, the agent will be found useful indeed. It seems especially to influence the orbital nerves; but has given great relief in cephalalgia, dysmenorrhoea, and general nephritic suffering. Dose of fluid extract, 30 drops to 1 fluid drachm three or four times a day.

RHAMNUS PURSHIANA.

CASCARA SAGRADA, SACRED RARK, CHITTEM, BEARBERRY.

This valuable article is a member of the buckthorn family. It is native to the Pacific Slope, where it is a small tree 20 to 30 feet high. Its young branches are woolly; leaves elliptical, 2 to 7 inches long, somewhat pubescent underneath; flowers large in clusters of 10 to 20; fruit black, ovoid, nearly half an inch long.

Cascara bark contains a brown, bitter resin freely soluble in alcohol and sparingly in water; a red and a light yellow resin; a fat oil and a volatile oil; some tannin, a crystallizable body and other elements. The species of R. frangula, native to the same section and formerly gathered indiscriminately with the R. purshiana, does not yield the same constituents.

Medical Properties.-The bark is most intensely bitter. Although long known as a medicine among the Indians and Spaniards of the Pacific Coast, the indefatigable Dr. J. H. Bundy first introduced it to the profession. Like many other new things, it had much opposition at first; but its merits finally secured it full recognition. Very few modern agents are so worthy of a first place with the profession.

Cascara bark is a tonic combining stimulating and relaxing properties, acting slowly and persistently, extending its influence through the alimentary canal and upon the gall duct's. The small intestines receive the larger share of its influence. It gently increases the mucous and glandular secretions of the bowels and gall ducts, promotes peristaltic movements, and leaves a toned condition with permanency of secretion and action. Such remedial influences are of great importance in a large number of cases; and no other one article, with the exception of euonymus, fills this particular line of requirements, and even that superb remedy is not so potent as cascara as an intestinal tonic.

It secures laxative results from the bowels, with steady excretion of bile, the stools being softened with intestinal secretions. It rarely causes griping, neither is it a mere cathartic or temporary evacuant; and while there are many more active cathartics, its efficacy in regulating and toning the bowels in chronic constipation is the most valuable quality of cascara. It also improves intestinal digestion; and thus, as well as removing from the intestinal tract the debris that so often poisons by resorption, cascarij promotes the general welfare of the system. In this way it is sometimes of much service in rheumatism and in syphilis; in haemorrhoids, by sustaining the portal circulation and emptying the liver; and is a good adjunct to tonics for dyspepsia, and to berberis and other hepatics in torpid liver. Dose of the fluid extract, 5 to 10 or 20 drops two or three times a day. Best given before meals in company with adjuvants; and it is often well to precede it by a saline cathartic.
It has been found that the bitter principle is not necessary to its laxative power; and now there is prepared an Aromatic Cascara, equal in potency to the fluid extract, nearly devoid of its intense bitterness, and made acceptable by the addition of aromatics.

RHUS AROMATICA.

FRAGRANT SUMACH, SWEET SUMACH.

Rhus glabra, the common sumac, is well known for the astringency of its leaves and bark, and the subacid astringency of its berries. From the severely poisonous characters of R. toxicodendron, R. venenata, R. radicans and R. pumila, it is often considered that all the rhus genus except the glabra are poisonous. Such is not the case, for R. aromatica is certainly not poisonous in any degree, if a multitude of careful clinical observers are to be credited.

Rhus aromatica is a shrub 2 to 5 feet high, of straggling growth, common in thickets east of the Rockies from Canada southward. Leaves three-parted, downy beneath when young, becoming smooth; leaflets 1 to 2 inches long, sessile, lateral ones ovate, terminal one rhomboid, giving a pleasant aroma when crushed. Flowers small, in clustered spikes, yellow, appearing in the spring before the leaves. Fruit a small drupe, crimson, covered with red and acid hairs. It is readily distinguished from the R. venenata, a shrub of much larger size having 7 to 13 leaflets, bearing very small green flowers and greenish white berries. See under R. toxicodendron in the latter part of the volume.

Medical Properties.-The bark of the root is nervine tonic with goodly astringent properties. Its principal action is upon the urinary organs, to which it is soothing and strengthening. For eneuresis it has been found of exceptional value, allaying the vesical sensitiveness and giving tone to the muscular structures.
Numerous reports of cases show it to be effective in that troublesome weakness, effecting an early cure in most patients. When it has failed, the cases seem to have required an addition of some such general tonic as scutellaria. It is a desirable associate of agrimony, epigea and other agents of this kind.

Rhus has also been used to advantage in diabetes insipidus, reducing decidedly the excessive urination. This fact has been observed frequently, and utilized to satisfaction; and it suggests a larger range of mild action on the nervous system than has usually been accorded to it. This property, together with its astringency, makes it useful in diarrhrea with spasmodic suffering; also in passive hemorrhages and in dysuria. As an agent of moderate power, it occupies a desirable place in the medicamenta, and deserves more thorough investigation. Dose of fluid extract, 10 to 30 drops four times a day, or 5 to 10 drops every three or two hours, when needed.

SABBATIA ELLIOTTII.

QUININE FLOWER.

A member of the gentian family common to pine barrens in our southeastern states. An herb about 2 feet high, much branched, bearing white flowers half an inch in length. Sabbatia belongs to a family distinguished for tonic properties, and sustains the gentian reputation. It enjoys a deserved reputation as an appetizer; and as an antiperiodic in malarial troubles is worthy of consideration. In like manner the better known Sabbatia angularis deserves more attention than it has received.

S. campestris has lilac flowers, and is common from Arkansas southward. In addition to its tonic properties it is reputed to be excellent in sick headache, probably from its invigorating influence upon the stomach and gall ducts. All these agents, as well as many of the gentians, contain a relaxing property and act persistently on the gall ducts; aiding to depurate the liver and remove general biliousness. It is probably in large measure because of this that they are so useful in intermittents.

SALIX.
WI LLOW.

Many of the willows have been used in medicine, particularly the S. alba and S. nigra. The bark of the trunk and root is employed, the former being the more astringent and the latter more tonic. In domestic practice they hold a good reputation; but their active principle, salicin, is the article now chiefly used by the profession. Salicin is a crystalline, white and bitter powder, soluble in 20 parts of cold water and less than 1 part of boiling water; less soluble in alcohol. It is a good tonic, stimulating the circulation somewhat, promoting intestinal rather more than gastric digestion, leaving the mucous surface with diminished secretions. It is useful in languid conditions, and for tonic purposes in general may be added to most alterative compounds, and to preparations designed for laxity of the female organs. In malarial troubles it may take the place of quinine; and while not such a potent antiperiodic, it does not cause the unpleasant cerebral symptoms of quinia salts. It has been customary to advise doses of 10 to 20 grains, but my experience prefers doses of 1 to 3 grains; and one-fourth to one-half a grain is often best.

Salicylic acid may be prepared from salicin by fusion with potassa hydrate; and out of this fact grew the thought that salicin must have the same properties as salicylic acid. The conclusion is made upon unsound chemical thoughts; for a substance of organic origin, when made to yield new compounds by chemical manipulation, need not be expected to transmit its properties to the new substance, nor should it be estimated by the qualities belonging to the new substance. In making claims of this kind for any substance, chemical science violates one of its own most common facts; and therapeutics should not be made to suffer on such unstable conceptions. Salicin in no degree or form resembles salicylic acid in its action. Some importance has been attached to a fluid extract of the catkins of Salix nigra as a calmative to excessive sexual desires, and a number of reports have been made in its favor. I have tried it in a number of cases, and the results have been uniformly nothing.

SANTALUM ALBUM.
SANDAL WOOD, WHITE SAUNDERS.

Red saunders wood has long been used as a pleasant flavoring and coloring material in pharmacy. Latterly the white, and also the yellow saunders (S. myrtifolium), have been used in perfumery and in medicine, because of their agreeable volatile oil.

This oil has obtained repute for its mildly stimulating action on mucous surfaces, especially on the genito-urinary organs; and has proven of value in sub-acute gonorrhea, also in sub-acute vaginitis. It is spoken of as a substitute for copaiba; but is by no means so resinous as the latter article, is of a milder grade of action, and is more acceptable to the stomach. These qualities make it an acceptable and effective agent, slightly increasing urination. It may be given alone in capsules, 3 to 5 drops three times a day; or it may be combined in varying proportions with copaiba, or with copaiba and oil of cubebs. Cinnamon makes it more palatable. Recently it has been combined with the saw palmetto. A fluid extract is prepared.

Apart from its action on the genito-urinary organs, sandal is a warming stimulant expectorant and antispasmodic in coughs, chronic bronchitis, etc.; and has proven of much service in the latter malady.

SERENOA SERRULATA.
SAW PALMETTO.

Sabal serrulata. A creeping, branching shrub palmetto, with stems six to eight feet long, bearing great fan-shaped leaves with saw-like edges, common in the" scrub forests" along the coasts from South Carolina to Florida. It bears a black, ovoid fruit, a true drupe generally spoken of as a berry. This fruit is much relished by stock, which fatten rapidly upon it. It contains a fixed and a volatile oil and resins; in which reside their medical qualities.

Medical Properties.-Saw palmetto berries have a somewhat sweetish taste when first eaten; but afterwards are rather acrid and pungent. As a medicine they are of a peculiar and not pleasant warming, stimulating character, rather persistent, containing a little relaxing quality. The action of this agent is somewhat extensive. It influences the sensory and sympathetic nerve peripheries, the mucous membranes, and the reproductive organs of both sexes.

On the mucous structures it gives a sense of warmth and relief from distress through the respiratory passages, proving of much service in sub-acute and chronic bronchitis and laryngitis, in old coughs, coughs following measles, pneumonia, la grippe, etc. It loosens tenacious mucus and diminishes catarrhal expectoration, and corrects the offensiveness of certain bronchial discharges. As a stimulant to these structures, it has proven good in catarrhal and other aphonias, and nasal catarrh; and some have commended its use in asthma and whooping cough to promote speedy expectoration. Its value in laryngeal phthisis is questionable. By its stimulating virtues it sometimes improves appetite, but is not an agent that would usually be selected for that purpose; yet it evidently promotes nutrition, and persons taking it for some time manifestly increase in flesh. This seems to be effected largely through its soothing and sustaining influence on the nervous system.

A peculiar and the most valued influence of serenoa, is the fact that it increases the activity of the breasts, ovaries, testes and prostate; and leads to an increase of their size and function, Improving sexual strength without materially exciting sexual appetite. Hence it has been employed in atrophy of the prostate and testes, in impotence, for vesical debility, distressing and too frequent urination, and all similar weaknesses of the genito-renal organs. Reports in its behalf in all these connections are numerous and strong, and give this agent peculiar value in a vexatious class of troubles. J. G. Rickenbacker, M. D., Orangeburg, S. C., writes me warmly on the article and its uses, and says: " A large portion of its power is expended upon the ganglionic nerves, and it seem;,; to be through this channel that the peculiar and valuable vitalizing action of the remedy upon the glands of the reproductive organs is obtained. The drug possesses the power of correcting faulty nutrition of these organs to a remarkable degree."

Serenoa is a potent agent. Pseudo-narcotic powers have been attributed to it; but I have seen nothing approaching narcotic action in the relief it gives the sensory nerves by sustaining them. It is so intense that it should be given with milder agents and with relaxing aromatics. The dose should be small, as 5 to 10 drops of fluid extract; but some give a drachm.

SIMABA CEDRON.

CEDRON.

A slender tree native to the tropics of South America, allied to quassia. Its fruit is a large drupe containing a single seed, this seed or almond being the medicinal portion of the plant.

Medical Properties.-Cedron seed is a bitter tonic with stimulating powers, and expends its chief influence on the nervous system from the centers outwardly. The bitterness is intense. Among the people it is used largely in the treatment of malaria; and some physicians who have tested it consider it a reliable antiperiodic in all intermit tents, more effective than quinine.

It stimulates the circulation by way of the nervous system, giving strength to the heart action and reducing its frequency when making the hurried struggle of depression. This power makes it a valuable agent in heart failure and general nervous prostration, in convalescence from typhoid, chronic diarrhea and atonic dyspepsia. By strongly sustaining the nervous centers it has proven of service in snake bites and other poisoned conditions. I have used it as a tonic in preparations designed for female weaknesses, and have been well pleased with its power to sustain the nerve tone; and have felt satisfied that it is a deserving remedy in impotence.

Cedron seed is a potent agent, requiring but a small dose. Its intense bitterness makes it preferable to use the seed or the solid extract in pill; but the fluid extract may be used, 1 to 3 drops every four hours.

SMILAX PSEUDO-CHINA.

VIRGINIA SARSAPARILLA, BAMBOO BRIAR, CHINA ROOT, CHINA BRIAR.

From Virginia southward and westward this plant is more or less common in open woods. It has a tuberous root of the lily character. The round stem, rising 2 to 5 feet, has on its lower part numerous sharp black prickles, which are wanting on the branches. Leaves 3 to 5 inches long. round-ovate, thin, green on both sides, bristly along the margins, 5-nerved. Berries black, 3-seeded.

Medical Properties.-Bamboo briar has long been popular among whites and negroes in the south as an alterative. It is moderately stimulating and somewhat tonic, acting gently but steadily upon the secreting organs, and especially on the skin and kidneys. For scrofulous swellings and ulcers, and skin diseases in general, it is an excellent remedy; and is esteemed highly among the blacks in syphilitic eruptions of the primary and secondary class.

Professional experience has confirmed these opinions of the people, and given the native bamboo briar a standing at least equal to that of Honduras sarsaparilla. It has been well spoken of in rheumatism. Combinations including it are numerous. One of its noted combinations is that known as McDade's formula, or McDade's alterative compound. It consists of 4 parts each bamboo briar, stillingia, burdock and poke roots, and one part xanthoxylum. Dr. McDade obtained it from the negroes, and the late Prof. J. Marion Sims urged it on the profession with his forceful enthusiasm. It is improved by leaving out the questionable poke root. Dose of bamboo briar fluid extract, 20 to 40 drops.

SOLIDAGO ODORA.

SWEET-SCENTED GOLDEN ROD.

At one time this plant was officinal in the U. S. Pharmacopoeia, as S. virgaurea was held in esteem by the Dublin College; but both were dropped out, and their places occupied by less desirable agents. Our country has about 50 species of Solidago, many of them very abundant in all sections; all except one bearing bright yellow flowers; some of them having furrowed, others angular and yet others round stems. Of them all, the S. odora is the only one that has medicinal properties of any particular value. Native to our land, it should receive the professional attention it deserves.

Solidago odora is from 18 inches to 3 feet high, having a little yellowish tone to its green color. Stem round, slender, with lines of down. Leaves 1 1/2 to 3 inches long, by about half an inch wide, pointed, with one strong yellowish midvein, but no veinlets; and by this vein, and also by a number of pellucid dots in the leaves, the odora is readily distinguished from other golden rods. The leaves are aromatic, and yield a fragrant yellowish-green oil by distillation. The flowers are in racemes 2 to 3 inches long, arranged in a simple row of small heads along the upper side.

Medical Properties.-The leaves are aromatic, diffusively stimulant and slightly relaxant. They are a warming and prompt carminative, useful in flatulence, and flatulent indigestion, and may be used as adjuncts to other remedies. In warm infusion they favor diaphoresis and sustain a good outward circulation. In recent suppression of the menses they serve a good purpose; and make a desirable addendum to preparations for dysmenorrhoea and amenorrhoea, relieving spasmodic suffering and promoting the menstrual flow, also somewhat increasing the amount of urine. An antiseptic property is reputed to belong to them, and this is said to be almost a specific for diphtheria when the article is used as a spray and exhibited inwardly. While a certain amount of real benefit from it as a diffusive stimulant is obtained, my own experience would not lead me to depend on it in that malady, much less to rely on it as an antiseptic. Dose of fluid extract, 10 to 40 drops.

SORGHUM SACCHARATUM.

BROOM CORN.

The article here referred to is the broom corn of the northern and western states, which furnishes the sorghum syrup. Its seeds have some demulcent properties, coupled with a mild diuretic and nervine tonic power. They act well in improving the flow of urine, and relieving irritability of the bladder and urethra. In sub-acute and chronic vesical catarrh they have been employed to advantage; and they give enough tone to the vesical structures to be of distinct service when micturition is too frequent and when it awakens elderly persons too often during the night. An humble agent, little known to the profession, the article will, I am sure, fully repay investigation. Its action is mild, and its field apparently limited; but I feel confident that it deserves careful attention. In infusion it may be used freely; or the fluid extract given in doses of half a drachm to a drachm.

STIGMATA MAIDIS.

CORN SILK.

For some years the silk of our common corn, Zea mays, has attracted professional attention as a diuretic. French physicians first used these stigmata-coming to America to find a remedy that we scorned to investigate, while we were going to the ends of the earth to find agents less valuable than many growing by our doors.

Corn silk has proven to be a mild stimulant with relaxant properties, slightly demulcent, quite agreeable to the taste. Its principal action is upon the renal organs, moderately increasing the secretion of urine, adding to the amount of solids eliminated and apparently aiding the solvency of phosphatic gravel.

Its action does not exhaust the kidneys, but gives them an improved tone. For acute renal congestion, cystitis, vesical catarrh, irritation of the urethra and neck of the bladder, and the distress incident to such conditions, it is one of our best agents. Prostatic irritation is benefited by it, and it will be found useful in irritable forms of spermatorrhoea; also in eneuresis, especially in combination with agrimony and capsella. From its soothing influence on the nervous system, I was led to combine it with polygonatum and similar agents in treating ovarian irritations and sub-acute uterine excitations, and with the happiest results, convincing me that it is a very desirable article in such connections and for spinal erethisms.

An infusion may be used freely. Dose of fluid extract, half a drachm to two drachms four or more times a day, drinking water freely.

STYLOSANTHES ELATIOR.

PENCIL FLOWER, AFTERBIRTH WEED.

A member of the family Leguminosre, and related to the bush clover, this little plant is frequent in the dry and barren woods from Long Island to Florida and westward to Arkansas. Its rigid little stems are about one foot high, branched, bearing trifoliate leaves, with dense pubescence on the side opposite the insertion of each leaf. The little yellow flowers are in clusters of 3 or 4 at the end of the branches, appearing in July and August.

Medical Properties.-Like many other agents that have secured favor with the profession, this herb has long been in use among the people and esteemed in domestic practice. Its position is that of an antispasmodic tonic, acting especially on the uterus, soothing it and relieving the suffering and crampings common to the latter weeks of pregnancy. False labor pains are quieted by it, threatening abortion generally averted, and strength sustained in labor. This humble plant deserves much confidence, for it exerts a power that is much needed and highly acceptable in medicine. An infusion may be used liberally every three hours; or the fluid extract given in doses of 10 to 20 drops. If its continued use is needed, three times a day is generally sufficient; and it may be given thus for two or three weeks prior to confinement.

SULPHUR.

It may seem needless to speak here of this ancient remedy, to which almost fabulous virtues were once attached; but it deserves to have especial attention called to it in some of its new curative relations. Reference is had to the washed and purified article called Sulphur lotum.

Sulphur has a peculiar local action in softening degenerated tissues and aiding in their removal. In diphtheria this is often of great advantage when ten to fifteen grains of the powder are blown in upon the membranous exudate from two to four times every twenty-four hours. Under this application the membrane usually exfoliates and is expelled promptly. In the first two days it may be used alone; hut after the second day it should be combined with an antiseptic, borax being sufficient for mild cases and myrrh being employed for those that are more severe. It has proven very efficient in this malady. Some physicians have employed it in diphtheria by giving ten to twenty gallons of it internally every two hours, and speak highly of its constitutional effects, as the agent is commonly absorbed and passes through the entire system. Applied to degenerate sores of any class it effectually removes all half-dead tissues, but leaves sound tissues unharmed and stimulated to a better granulating effort. By this action it soon cleanses away the decaying debris of foul ulcers, almost acting as a mild escharotic without in any sense being escharotic. I have thus used it with gratifying results on indolent and scrofulous ulcers, foul syphilitic sores, and even upon lupus and true carcinoma, till the removal of the offensive elements called for other applications. It may be dusted on in powder, or moderated by combining it with hydrastis, or with borax and hydrastis; or mixed with hydrastis and glycerine.

The fatal action of sulphur on certain parasites is well known, as in the case of scabies, a sulphur ointment soon removing that troublesome insect. A case of filariae sanguinis came under my notice, where a lady seemed to be alive with hair-like parasites half an inch to an inch in length. They came out through the skin, the mucous membrane of the mouth and nose, the conjunctivae, were half vomited in quantities, passed away in the urine, crept out of the vagina in dozens, creating intense irritation everywhere. All treatment seemed to be useless. At last sulphur was given in teaspoonful doses three times a day, and was soon followed by the discharge of masses of those parasites. In a few days they ceased to appear on the skin and elsewhere, the inflammation of the conjunctivae disappeared, appetite and digestion returned, and in a short time the lady regained her health.

I was consulted in a case of great hepatic distention, where the history and an exploration showed it to be hydatids. I advised sulphur in teaspoonful doses every morning for a week; then omit three mornings, and resume for another week, and thus on. The bowels, which had been obstinately constipated, began to move naturally in a few days, and soon to carry off large quantities of gelatinous-looking material. The patient was at a long distance from me, and I was dependent upon the attending physician for occasional reports, which were to the effect that the man improved steadily though slowly, gained in his digestion and general appearance, and after a few months the liver had returned to about its normal size. Little was used besides the sulphur, and some hydrastis as a tonic.

In some very intractable cases of moist eczema I have dusted the parts twice a day with a powder of sulphur four parts, gum camphor one part, starch ten to fifteen parts; and with very gratifying results. In dry eczema and other forms of crusting skin troubles, I have incorporated one part of sulphur with four or more parts of glycerite of starch, and have been more than satisfied with the results.

Sulphur being insoluble in water and alcohol, cannot be used externally in some cases where its application would be desirable, except as incorporated with a petroleum product. In a measure this difficulty may be overcome by using it in the new menstruum, Polysolve. This dissolves two percent of sulphur, and makes an oily application that is absorbable and non-irritative. Thus combined, sulphur is useful in removing dandruff and in the treatment of squamous syphilides. Sulphur soaps are familiar articles. Ichthyol and thiol are sulphur compounds, the latter being soluble.

TAKA-DIASTASE.

For the purpose of promoting the digestion of starch elements when the ptyalin of the saliva and the enzyme of the pancreas is deficient, diastase from malted grains has long been known as a potent agent. It has been utilized in various forms of malt preparations, obtained only by the germination of barley and other cereals under the influence of warmth and moisture. See Malt. A new process of developing diastase, and of obtaining it in more effective form, is claimed to have been discovered by Mr. Jokichi Takamine, of Japan. His process depends upon using a new ferment from the fungus Eurotium oryzae; and the product obtained after the several steps in manufacture has been named, in honor to its discoverer, Taka-diastase. It is a tasteless powder, odorless, pale yellow; and seems to act as well in acidulous as in alkaline secretions. It is claimed that it will quickly convert one hundred times its own weight of starch into a soluble state. The article thus becomes valuable in those numerous and very troublesome cases of dyspepsia where the use of bread, potatoes and other amylaceous foods causes bloating, acid eructations, loss of appetite and distress. My own use of it has brought very favorable results. Dose, two to five grains with the meal.

THIOLUM- THIOL.

This product was devised to replace the ill-smelling ichthyol. It is made by combining sulphur with hydrocarbons and then distilling. The thin, dark-brown neutral liquid distillate is Thiol. It has an odor similar to Russian leather, is miscible with water and glycerine, and makes a sulphur compound in soluble form. It is used for external applications in a large class of skin diseases, especially the different forms of moist and pustular eczema, chilblains in the ulcerative stage, scrofulous and syphilitic ulcers, recent effusions into joints, moist inflammatory processes, etc. The reports in its behalf are very satisfactory, its action seeming to be moderately antiseptic and distinctly drying to effusions and even hardening to the skin. It may be used as a liquid application diluted in any proportion with water, equal parts or 1 to 4; or with glycerine 1 to 9. The liquid thiol is dried and furnished as thiolum siccum, and this may be mixed with starch (1 to 4) and used as a dusting powder, or made into an ointment with vaseline and lanoline. The ointment is used on rheumatic joints.

THUJA OCCIDENTALIS.

AMERICAN ARBOR VITAE, TREE OF LIFE.

Among the evergreen shrubs, the arbor vitae holds a front rank. For some years its smaller branches with their appressed leaves have been used in medicine. They contain a volatile oil, resin, tannic acid and several indeterminate principles. It has been supposed that the oil was similar to that of savin, but there is no good ground for this.

Medical Properties.-As yet the literature on this agent is limited. It has in some hands given most desirable results in the treatment of cancer, condylomata, and other vicious growths. In cancer it is said to overcome the foul odor, relieve the acute suffering, reduce the deposits and finally effect a cure. Such good results have not been obtained by all practitioners; and as the testimony thus conflicts, there must be some additional knowledge needed. New information may show its adaptability to some cases and not to others. Dr. H. C. Noble reports its use in thirty cases of spermatorrhoea, with but . one failure; and some of its successes here are quite astonishing, if the reports are not too colored. In venereal vegetations its effects seem to be admirable. It is a stimulating astringent of decided power; and if further clinical observations prove its action to be sanative, and show its exact influence, it will no doubt become a valuable article. It has been used for suppressed menstrualtion, under the impression that it was similar to savine, and some have given it for rheumatism and intermittents, but this is very indefinite.

A saturated tincture is given in doses of half a drachm to a drachm two or three times a day, and at the same time applied locally. Dose of the fluid extract, 3 to 5 drops thrice daily.

TRIFOLIUM PRATENSE.

RED CLOVER.

Medical Properties.-Red clover blossoms are largely relaxant with a smaller portion of stimulation, mild in power and slow in action. Among the people they have long been used by infusion to arrest the paroxysms of whooping-cough, for which they are reported good; also as a wash for foul ulcers, and in solid extract to apply to cancers. It is, however, for their favorable influence upon the excreting organs that they are now most prized. They are an alterative of mild grade, opening the cutaneous glands, the bowels and the kidneys; for which they are useful in scrofula and cutaneous eruptions, and as an associate with such an agent as cascara in habitual constipation. Being mild and mostly relaxant, they should be combined with more stimulating and tonic alteratives, as Stillingia and rumex; and when thus associated, the trifolium makes a useful adjunct in the treatment of secondary syphilis. A Syrup of Trifolium Compound has been highly commended, containing trifolium, stillingia, arctium root, phytolacca root, berberis, picramnia, xanthoxylum, and potassium iodide. In this, trifolium replaces the bamboo-briar of McDade's formula, and the objectionable potassium iodide is added. I offer a much better combination for secondary syphilis, namely: Trifolium and ampelopsis, four parts each; stillingia, corydalis and berberis. aquifolium, two parts each; xanthoxylum bark, one part. I have used this formula liberally in my own practice, and am justified in urging it upon the attention of the profession for degenerate ulcers, scrofula and secondary syphilis-having known it to soften and remove gummata, without any use of the weakening potassium iodide. I name it Trifolium and Berberis Compound.

Dose of trifolium fluid extract, half a drachm to a drachm three or four times a day.

TRITICUM REPENS.

COUCH GRASS, QUITCH GRASS.

Couch grass belongs to the same genus as our edible wheat, Triticum vulgare. It is a common and very undesirable weed, its pointed rhizome creeping under the surface and producing a new plant at every severance between its joints. Lower portion of the culm trailing, bearing wheat-like spikes about three inches long.

Medical Properties.--Under the name Agropyrum, the root of this plant was a medicament among the ancients, and possibly was in use before the Christian era; but its virtues were obscured by the "craze" after mineral agents in the later centuries, and have but recently been rediscovered. It is quite demulcent, and like most demulcents acts on the kidneys and urinary passages. Connected with this is a gentle grade of stimulating property. It increases the flow of urine, relieves renal congestion, and soothes the vesical and urethral surfaces. For these purposes it is a serviceable article in a large class of sub-acute cases, including suppression of urine and calculous irritations. It has been pronounced capable of dissolving urinary calculi; but this is more than questionable, though its beneficial action on the renal secretion certainly diminishes the liability to enlargement of such accretions and favors the early expulsion of small deposits. It is a favorite among the people who drink freely of its decoction; and the profession is finding it meritorious.

TURNERA APHRODISIACA.

DAMIANA.

Damiana comes from Mexico, and allied species of similar medical properties from California and Central America. It is a small shrub-like plant, resembling a mint, with yellowish-white fragrant flowers.

Medical Properties.-Damiana leaves enjoyed a popular reputation among the Mexicans and Mexican Indians as a stimulus of the sexual appetite. From the people the article became known to the profession, and now holds a prominent place as an aphrodisiac. It is an aromatic stimulant with some tonic properties, not pleasant to the taste but quite warming, moderately diffusive in its action. Its principal impression is made upon the nervous centers, from whence it is distributed to the urinary and genital apparatus, exciting sexual desires and increasing the flow of urine. It also promotes the menstrual flow, and may relieve amenorrhoea; incites hepatic secretion, and may promote catharsis, and increases circulation.

For sexual impotence it is considered very reliable, as it stimulates and tones up the reproductive organs of both sexes. Probably it acts first and directly upon the basilar portion of the brain; but it also unquestionably influences the nerves and circulation of the genitalia. Leaving a tonic impression, it becomes of service in genital weaknesses, enlarged and painful prostate, etc. It seems also to act fairly well as a heart tonic. Extravagant statements have been given out concerning it, but the reliable reports in its favor are good.

Dose of the fluid extract, 20 to 30 drops three or four times a day; powdered extract of the leaves, 5 to 15 grains.

VACCINIUM CRASSIFOLIUM.
BILBERRY.

A member of the whortleberry (huckleberry) family, found in sandy bogs along the coast of the Southern States, allied to the V. vitis-idrea or cowberry. A shrubby plant with trailing stems 2 or 3 feet long, bearing small clusters of nearly white flowers in the axils of the little leaves. Fruit a small black berry.

Medical Properties.-The leaves of this plant are a tonic of the mildly astringent class, expending their influence mostly upon the genito-urinary organs. Resembling uva ursi in their action, they are much more diuretic than the latter, and always leave a toned condition. Such qualities give them distinct value in ascites and renal dropsy generally. In vesical catarrh and chronic cystitis the agent is an excellent one; also in gleet and as a wash in leucorrhrea. Combined with mitchella and polygonatum it is of service in lax conditions of the female organs; and with agrimony will be of service in eneuresis. It deserves a more prominent place than it has yet received among our native remedial agents.

VERNONIA FASCICULATA.
IRONWEED.

For several years I have been using the leaves of this gigantic plant of our country, and wish to offer my experience to the profession. Ironweed roots have been used by some for malarial troubles; but its leaves furnish us an astringent tonic of a truly desirable character, and one that is quite acceptable to the stomach when many other tonics are not well received. In those indigestions where the stomach is in a lax condition, with poor appetite, sense of epigastric heaviness after eating, flatulence, pyrosis, and a moderate atonic condition, it will be found of exceptional value. Also in diarrhoea from atonic indigestion, chronic diarrhrea, and similar lax states of the tissues. For local use in leucorrhoea it is good, not being a mere astringent but a tonic that acts most kindly on mucous surfaces. Growing nearly everywhere, lifting its showy purple flower-heads six to ten feet high from August to October, this plant is thoroughly deserving of professional attention. Its leaves must be dried quickly, else they will mildew. It is not, in the market among fluid extracts; but an infusion or mild tincture may be used. It is an admirable companion to the American columba, Frasera Cariolinensis.

VIBURNUM LANTANOIDES.
HOBBLE BUSH, MOOSEWOOD.

Canada, the New England states, and other northern sections are the habitats of this member of .the viburnum family. It is a shrub of two to five feet III height, with slender branches that often bend to the ground and take root as do trailing plants. Its leaves are very large, broadly oval, rather heart-shaped at the base, the strong veins on the under side closely studded with short brown hairs. Fruit red and finally purplish black. From its common name, moose wood, it is liable to be confounded with the Dirca palustris, or the Acer striatum, both of which receive the same name.

Medical Properties.-This agent is as yet practically unknown to the profession; but two members of its family, V. opulus and V. prunifolium, are already among our favorite agents, and offer a worthy introduction for this one. My attention was first called to it by the late Dr. A. C. De Brisay, of Petit Rocher, New Brunswick. He was himself suffering from severe bronchial irritation and cough, following a cold, and obtained decided relief from the soreness and the spasmodic cough by using an infusion of the small twigs, taking it freely. So prompt and marked was the benefit obtained, that he soon after wrote me and sent me a goodly supply to test. He knew it only by the common name of moosewood; and as he could send me only leaves and twigs, it was some time before I could determine it botanically.

Dr. De Brisay's kindness supplied me with a sufficient amount of the article to satisfy me as to its qualities and its worth. Subsequently I obtained larger supplies from Canadian friends; and from ample experience with it am now able to speak of it confidently. Its properties, as with the other viburni, lie in the bark; but the shrub is of such moderate size that the entire branches and twigs may be used. The bark is pleasantly bitter, and the medulla of the stems yields some demulcent. They are nervine and antispasmodic in action, peculiarly soothing to mucous surfaces and acceptable to the stomach, leaving a goodly tonic impression. Upon the air passages their action is prompt and effective, soothing the surfaces and allaying the spasmodic cough. Probably their chief influence is expended there, furnishing us a desirable remedy in all that class of coughs and bronchial troubles where an antispasmodic and mildly tonic medicament is needed. But I have also found the article quite useful in some nervous forms of indigestion, and acceptable to weak and irritable stomachs where more positive agents could not be used. In cases of uterine sensitiveness, with leucorrhcea and nervous irritability, I am confident it will be found of signal benefit.

VIBURNUM PRUNIFOLIUM.

BLACK HAW, AMERICAN SLOE.

Black haw is in that section of the cranberry and snowball family which bears drupaceous fruit of a dark purple or black color. It is a low and branching shrub at the north, but a slender tree of 20 feet or more in the south.

Medical Properties. -Twenty-five years ago I wrote on the medical virtues of black-haw hark, pronouncing it worthy of more thorough employment; and the virtues I then attributed to it have been confirmed fully by later investigations. Bark from the root is preferable. but that from the trunk possesses the same qualities. Like V. opulus, it is a soothing tonic with a goodly measure of astringency; and is found to contain a small amount of viburnin, some valerianic acid, tannin, and a bitter resinous matter. It acts largely on the nervous system, allaying excitement, proving notably antispasmodic, and imparting healthy tone. The uterus receives the larger share of its influence; and probably we have no medicine that will so reliably quiet the erethisms of this organ, arrest threatened abortion, and correct menorrhagia and other uterine hemorrhages. Where there have been miscarriages and a repetition is apprehended, or where untoward circumstances endanger such a loss of the foetus, black haw will rarely fail to relieve the excitement and spasmodic contractions of the uterus, and carry gestation forward naturally.

Its moderate astringing power acts well in closing the bleeding vessels, and increases the virtue of the article in too free or too frequent menstruation. It will be found useful in diarrhoea with spasmodic sufferings; and, like many nervine tonics, will increase the renal flow in cases where the nervous system is largely at fault. As I pointed out twenty years ago, many cases of diabetes and albuminuria have no small degree of their pathology starting from the spinal nervous system, and this particular viburnum is an admirable agent to correct such conditions and benefit those renal diseases. For these purposes it may be combined with viburnum opulus, and a portion of scutellaria; and a similar combination is of great service in the entire list of hysteric and neur-asthenic conditions. Nearly all the uses of black haw have been in the uterine dangers above mentioned, and its value there cannot be questioned; but an equally large satisfaction will he obtained from using it in these nerve conditions, and in dysmenorrhoea, to soothe general "nervous excitement, aid better sleep, etc. Generally it is used in form of fluid extract, of which the dose is from 20 drops to half a fluid drachm three or four times a day. It may be given every hour or two hours, till relief has been obtained. In habitual miscarriage its use should be commenced a month before the time of anticipated danger, and several days before the period in profuse menstruation. Its taste may be disguised by a little cinnamon, which also aids in checking a tendency to flowing. It can be added to compound mitchella to much advantage.

VERBENA URTICOEFOL[A.

WHITE VERVAIN.

In 1869 I called the attention of the profession to this article, and to its companion, V. hastata. blue vervain. I considered them agents of decided power and deserving of professional attention as tonic hepatics in biliousness and intermittents. A few others have confirmed my opinion; but the two articles still remain comparatively unknown to physicians, perhaps ignored because so very common everywhere, perhaps too bitter to be attractive. Probably this hitterness may be separated from the other properties of the plants, as has been done with cascara sagrada.

It is my belief, from no small or uncertain experience, that these articles are almost or quite the equals of cascara for giving tone to the hepatic organs and the smaller intestines. Slow but steady in action, they promote the secretion and expulsion of bile, increase peristalsis and intestinal digestion, and leave a tonic impression that is desirable. This action adapts them to hepatic torpor and its long train of sequences, to malarial troubles and to chronic constipation. In rheumatic cases with biliousness, they are good to remove the cholaemic conditions; and are useful in jaundice and in hepatic dropsy. The white variety acts upon the uterus in amenorrhoea, tardy labor pains and similar troubles, especially if aided by warm applications to the extremities and the surface. It promises to prove an admirable agent in this relation. Dose, fluid extract of leaves, 10 to 20 drops as often as needed.

VERBASCUM THAPSIS.

MULLEIN.

The leaves of this common plant are by no means new to medicine. I have heretofore written of them as valuable to promote absorption of dropsical and other effusions; thoroughly soothing to the nervous system, whether used inwardly or outwardly; and useful in diarrhoea and other excessive discharges. They deserve far more recognition than they have received: Mullein oil, obtained from the flowers by exposing them to the sun in a bottle and finally expressing them, has come into use for deafness. Strong commendations have been given to the article in this connection; but nothing definite has been stated as to the particular forms of deafness to which it is suited. It is an exceedingly soothing and lubricating article, and undoubtedly merits attention. It is to be suspected, however, that some oil of mullein on the market is only a strong tincture with a goodly portion of glycerine added. That would be of small value in deafness.

PART II.

AGENTS THAT ARE TOXIC.

THE BASIS OF CLASSIFICATION.

In this part is classed a series of articles that are more or less toxic in their properties. They are agents which are used to effect the relief of certain specified symptoms, without securing an improvement of the pathological conditions underlying those symptoms. And in promoting that relief, their action is often quite uncertain and unreliable; they disturb the physiological conditions; and their administration cannot be pressed incautiously, lest their use be followed by serious or even fatal consequences.

By these facts the toxicity of these articles is determined. In my judgment, these facts do not warrant the use of any of these agents in the treatment of disease, inasmuch as they do not restore the normal or physio-logical status, but promote the development of new pathological conditions. It seems to me that the remarkable feeling of unrest and dissatisfaction everywhere observable in the profession, is due largely to the succession of disappointments following upon the use of toxic agencies. One list after another is presented, is found untrust-worthy, and is put aside only to open the way for another list that soon proves equally unsatisfying.

Can we hope to establish Therapeutics as a settled science, except as we turn from a line of thought that has not established it, and proceed to develop a truly non-toxic medicamenta, as was the hope of the Fathers of Medicine in the past centuries?

While seeking to add my mite in this line of investigation, the later toxic agents are here presented and both sides of the reports given in a spirit of fairness. Every new article is not described; for many of them are too recent to have a standing; and many are merely commercial offerings protected hy letters patent, and have no higher place than secret proprietary medicines.

AILANTHUS GLANDULOSA. Tree of Heaven, Chinese Sumach.

Ailanthus trees are common in our cities and towns, cultivated for their rapid growth. The bark has been commended as a germicide, and is said to destroy the round worm and the tape worm. It purges rather actively, but seems only occasionally to prove anthelmintic. It is quite poisonous. often exciting emesis with much prostration, vertigo and cold sweats.

ANDIRA ARAROBA. Goa Powder, Chrysarobin, Chrysophanic Acid.

Andira is a stately leguminous tree of Brazil; and from large clefts in its wood is obtained a yellowish or brown powder called Goa. By treating this with benzol, its yellow active principle is obtained, termed chrysarobin. When this is given inwardly, it undergoes oxidation at the expense of the blood, and chrysophanic acid is produced; and this is expelled by the urine, causing severe irritation, albuminuria, and even bloody urine. Chrysarobin and goa powder are used as ointments with vaseline for psoriasis, eczema, ringworm and other cutaneous affections. It is absorbed freely by the skin and converted into chrysophanic acid, causing the kidney disturbances just named. Applied about the face or near the genitals, it is apt to cause oedema of these parts. It is an exceedingly harsh article, causes burning and irritation, stains the sound skin deeply, and the local affections said to be cured by it soon return.

AMYL NITRITE.

By the action of nitric or nitrous acid on amylic alcohol, amyl nitrite is produced. A yellowish and clear liquid, with a fruity odor and taste, volatile, inflammable, insoluble in water.

It acts on the body with great rapidity, and is usually given by inhalation, 3 to 5 drops on a handkerchief being held over the nose and mouth till it begins to cause flushing of the face and hurried action of the heart. A few drops in a thin shell of glass are called "pearls," and one of these is crushed in the handkerchief for use. Occasionally the agent is given internally, dropped on sugar. It has been used for spasms, as epilepsy, asthma, tetanus, hysterical convulsions and angina pectoris. It is strongly toxic, and doubly dangerous because of its great rapidity of action. A small quantity in a few moments will arouse most excessive beating of the heart. intense flushing of the face, and such a violent crowding of blood to the head as to give a sensation of bursting. While pulse frequency is so greatly increased, the force of the circulation is diminished. It greatly depresses the spinal centres, causes progressive loss of reflex power and of muscular strength, and experiments on dogs caused death from failure of respiration.

ANEMONE PULSATILLA. Pasque Flower, Pulsatilla.

Pulsatilla, a European anemone, has been much used by some physicians as a stimulant and anodyne to the uterine organs, in amenorrhoea and nervous dysmenorrhoea, neuralgic headache, hysteria, nervous debility, nasal and bronchial catarrh, and secondary syphilis. While some praise it in these wide fields, others disparage it. Dose. of tincture, 3 to 10 drops; of fluid extract, 1 to 3 drops. Full doses frequently cause vesicular and pustular eruptions. Anemonine, its active principle, is in white, odorless crystals. This diminishes cardiac activity and voluntary movements by depressing the spinal centres; and dyspncea, torpor, paralysis of the limbs, diarrhoea, headache, and death by cardiac paralysis.

ANTIFEBRIN. Acetanilid, Phenyl-acetanimide.

Obtained by boiling aniline in glacial acetic acid. In white, inodorous crystals, slightly tart, soluble in 194 parts of cold water and 5 of alcohol. It is the most popular of the coal-tar derivatives, given extensively as an antipyretic; as an analgesic in rheumatism, neuralgias, headache and all sufferings, and for epilepsy.

It is distinctly toxic. Dr. V on Goldman calls it "a treacherous remedy." It depresses the spinal cord and bulb, and produces vaso-motor disturbances. Very small doses frequently cause "weak heart, symptoms of depression, hyperidrosis, chilliness;" also "cyanosis, cardiac depression and collapse." It enters the circulation and "the state of the blood is considerably modified, whence the lowering of temperature produced by it." In usual doses it is liable to cause drenching perspiration, notable cyanosis, and often profound collapse. Its full action produces "stupor, prostration, hesitating movements, cyanosis, irregular pulse, analgesia, collapse, a series of convulsive shocks, and death." It is this drug that druggists so freely dispense as "headache powders," to the great detriment of the public. Marked cyanosis and collapse have followed its absorption when dusted on wounds, sores, burns and eczema.

Antikamnia is a proprietary medicine said to be made of acetanilid, caffeine and soda bicarb. If so, the combination delays and partly conceals the acetanilid; but presently its treachery is revealed, and "mild cyanosis" and "mild collapse" frequently follow. Several other proprietary compounds contain acetanilid.

ANTIPYRIN. Parodyn, Phenazon.

One of the earliest of the coal-tar derivatives, in colorless-crystals readily soluble in water and alcohol. Used chiefly to lower the temperature in fever. Acts rapidly, beginning to show its antipyretic effect in less than an hour, with profuse cold sweating. These results are due to its toxic depression of the spinal cord and nervous system. Dr. Cauquil, Paris, says: "Its action is transient; and if it diminishes fever, with the greater part of the inconveniences which the latter brings, it remains absolutely ineffectual against the disease itself." "Ordinary doses cause languor, depression, exhausting and almost colliquative perspiration, lividity; often violent urticaria, erythema and general dermatitis with oedema; dyspnoea, hysterical restlessness, and other severe constitutional symptoms. Larger doses induce vertigo, agonizing headache, trembling, distress at the heart, increased pulse, sub-normal temperature; and then usually deep coma, stertor, dilated pupils, epileptiform convulsions, collapse." It depresses the cortex of the brain and the spinal nerves, produces paralysis of the motor and sensory nerve trunks, diminishes the urine and quickly loads the blood with urea. Recently lauded to the highest, it is now almost abandoned.

ASPIDOSPERMA QUEBRACHO-BLANCO. Quebracho.

Quebracho is an evergreen tree belonging to the family of apocynacaee. The bark has been introduced to medicine for the relief of asthma and other forms of difficult breathing; and for pneumonia.
Reports concerning its usefulness have been very warm, the fluid extract being given in doses of 15 to 40 drops several times a day.

It has repeatedly been noticed that its prolonged use, or its exhibition in considerable quantity, is likely to be attended with unpleasant consequences. Among these is a severe dyspnroea-the very trouble that it is especially used for. It causes the pulse to sink rapidly, sometimes reducing it to 20 per minute, effecting this result through cardiac innervation. It relieves dyspnoea by a similar direct action upon the nerves governing respiration, causing their depression, and finally so reducing their power as to cause the secondary dyspnoea above alluded to. The respirations are less deep than natural, and the blood is changed in color similar to that caused by poisoning with carbonic oxide. Experiments with it on lower animals caused dyspnoea, motor palsy, and death by asphyxia.

BRUNFELSIA HOPEANA. Manaca, Vegetable Mercury.

Manaca is a branching shrub indigenous to tropical South America, with smooth and thick leaves, and fragrant bluish flowers. Natural order Solanaceae. Manaca root has been introduced to medicine as an anti-syphilitic and anti-rheumatic, and a general alterative.

Enthusiastic reports of its curative powers have been given, and by some it has been thought a specific for rheumatism, while the title of Vegetable Mercury intimates their opinion of it in the treatment of syphilis.

Experiments with it upon animals present the following results: Early restlessness, piteous crying, constant walking, gait soon becoming trembling and unsteady; respiration reduced to one-third or less, pulse reduced nearly one-half; tenacious saliva running from the mouth abundantly. Presently there come twitchings of the legs and jaws, inability to stand, dilatation of the pupils, general clonic spasms with labored respiration from spasms of the chest and diaphragm. Consciousness remains intact, while power of locomotion and co-ordination is lost; thus showing its intense toxic action to be on the spinal cord, from which center it extends to the heart and respiratory apparatus, depressing or destroying two-thirds their force until death ensues. After death, the heart is found dilated, flabby, and containing fluid blood on both sides; the lungs are congested, the stomach and intestines filled with tenacious and frothy mucus. Corresponding effects are produced by it on man.

CHLORALAMID. Formidate of Chloral.

Chloral amid is produced by the interaction between chloral and formamide. In colorless and shining crystals, of a bitter taste, soluble in 20 parts of cold water and in 1 1/2 parts strongest alcohol. Alkalies decompose it into its original constituents of chloral and formamide; and it is thus gradually decomposed by tbe alkalinity of the blood, so that the chloral acts a little at a time as the separation proceeds.

It is used almost wholly for the purpose of procuring sleep in insomnia due to nervousness, hysteria, cardiac disease, and alcoholic excesses; but is not often effectual when there is sharp suffering, for it does not relieve suffering. Usually it begins to act in from one to two hours; and may continue ten or more hours, as the chloral is little by little set free in the blood. Its action is in all respects the same as chloral, though milder and also less constant, often failing. Its principal effect is upon the cerebral cortex, which it depresses, thereby causing sleep; in a smaller degree upon the spine, which it also depresses. In therapeutic doses of 30 to 45 grains, about two-thirds of which is chloral, it is liable to be followed by vertigo, nausea, thirst, dryness of the mouth, loss of appetite and general deficiency of the secretions. Frequently it causes headache and mental confusion, continuing for many hours; and in susceptible persons or full doses it has produced cardiac weakness, rapid and feeble pulse and restlessness which necessitated forcible restraint, as also severe giddiness and symptoms of intoxication with great excitement.-Dr. Patterson in Lancet, October, 1889.

COLA ACUMINATA. Kola, Soudan Coffee, Ooora.

Cola is a tree of much beauty, native to Western Africa, now cultivated in the East and West Indies and South America. It has a smooth round trunk, green bark, and oval leaves nearly a foot in length. Leaves thick, leathery, smooth; flowers numerous, in cymose panicles; fruit yielding from 5 to 12 nuts or seeds in each carpel. These nuts are variously red and white, and weigh from a drachm to an ounce or more.

Kola nuts have attracted much attention as a stimulant strongly resembling coffee. The Portuguese found the African natives using them, and followed their example; whence Dutch and English traders became interested, and the trade in kola nuts has become considerable.

Extravagant reports were made of the power of kola to sustain the muscular and nervous systems under fatigue, the eating of a few nuts supporting travelers on long journeys almost without food, imparting strength to the laborer, preventing loss of wind in the runner or the mountain climber, and quenching thirst. Held in esteem among the natives, they became luxuries among the rich and were costly articles of commerce one and two centuries ago.

Since the introduction of kola to the civilized world, the commercial praises of the article have been as extravagant as those used by the wild Africans; and possibly more extravagant by the degree to which civilized language surpasses uncivilized. When carefully sifted, the facts seem to be that kola is a stimulant that for a time renders one capable of sustaining an unusual fatigue, and gives a sense of invigoration. It is used by the natives as we use coffee; but its more common use is by masticating the nut, keeping it in the month continually and swallowing the saliva.

Medicinally it has been commended for nervous weariness, cardiac weakness, diarrhoea, dyspepsia, and during convalescence. While it sustains, it also notably diminishes waste; and while it energetically stimulates the cardiac contractions, it has a paralyzing effect upon striated muscles in full doses. It increases the amount of water passed through the kidneys, but reduces the solids and especially lessens the extractives cast out by the urine. From this it is urged that the article sustains by saving aliment that otherwise would undergo change and be passed off as urea. In other words, kola retards the processes of alimentation. and causes to be retained the waste elements that are liberated by exertion, at the same time causing a feeling of exhilaration. This is not a physiological action, but an interference with the ordinary functions of the body. Alcohol retains the waste elements; and hence was claimed to be a saver of food and a sustainer of strength, precisely as is now claimed for kola. So far as observation has determined, the article is an excitant, not unlike alcohol in some respects, though lacking the stupefying power of the latter. Its use too much resembles the use of strong drink, and needs to be guarded against rather than encouraged among the people. Some of its compounds are little better than excuses for tippling.

CONVALLARIA MAJALIS. Lily of the Valley.

This is the little garden lily so loved for its white and fragrant flowers. The flowers, as also the leaves and roots (rhizomes), have been used in medicine, and by some have been valued for an apparent tonic action on the heart; also as being actively diuretic, and hence serviceable in dropsy of cardiac origin. Ii is said to calm and strengthen the heart in palpitations, giving it more force and regularity; and hence useful in conditions with feebleness and irregularity of action, especially in mitral obstruction. It contains two active principles: one, convallarin, is soluble in alcohol and not in water; the other, convallarnarin, is readily soluble in both water and alcohol. An infusion contains the latter principle; a fluid extract commonly contains both principles.

Experience has shown these active principles to be vigorously poisonous, the convallamarin being the more intense and rapid. Dr. H. Marme, Germany, gave the following results of his investigations: "Convallarin, in doses of 3 or 4 grains, acts as a purgative. Convallamarin, even in small doses, produces active vomiting, and acts especially on the heart, at first diminishing- the number of pulsations, afterwards rendering them more frequent, and causing death in a few minutes. The heart appears to be paralyzed, and cannot be excited after death." His experiments were on animals. Dr. Leubuscher found it caused progressive paralysis, at first with cramp-like tremblings and finally complete loss of reflex activity, death occurring- in from half to three-quarters of an hour, from systolic cardiac arrest. A marked feature before the arrest of the heart is great derangement in its rhythm, the regular contraction of ventricle and auricle being completely destroyed. Convallamarin acts through the vagi, and reduces heart activity in the line of paralysis.

CREASOTUM. Creasote.

Creasote is obtained by distilling wood-tar, and is an old-time agent of well-known poisonous powers. Recently it has been brought into prominence by a more refined product being distilled from beechwood; which is commended very earnestly as an antiseptic in all offensive sores and maladies, and very especially as a remedy in erysipelas and typhoid fever. It is claimed for it that it will speedily abort the latter malady, and render it simple and easily curable. Its action is really but little different from that of carbolic acid, the same in kind though milder in power. Toxic doses cause dizziness, dimness of sight, lethargy, diminished heart action, convulsions and coma. The New York Medical Journal for July 28, 1896, quotes from foreign journals a case in which a woman with bronchitis took three doses as prescribed; and it speedily caused difficulty of swallowing, vomiting, diarrhea, anaesthesia and paralysis about the tongue and palate, albumen and hyaline casts in the urine, and death from collapse in four days.

CREOLIN, Cresol.

The cresols and the cresylic acids, of which there arc three isomerides, are homologues of carbolic acid, and are obtained by the fractional distillation of the coal-tar oil that comes over between 375° and 410° F. They have a very strong odor of creasote, are insoluble in water, and are similar in toxic action to carbolic acid but less powerful. By the addition of soap they are rendered soluble, and are used thus in forming creolin, lysol, phenolin, etc.; and form soluble cresylates with an alkali.

Creolin is an emulsion or cresol with a resinous soap. It is used mostly for antiseptic purposes, being diluted largely, as 5 parts to the 1000; and sometimes one part to the thousand is sufficiently strong to use in washing sores and injecting into cavities. Such dilute solutions are used by some in fermentative diarrhoea, cholera morbus, etc. A five per cent. ointment on vaseline has been used for scabies. Employed outwardly or inwardly, it causes toxic symptoms; among the most common of which are nausea, restlessness, faintness and amblyopia.

DUBOISIA MYOPOROIDES. Duboisia.

This plant belongs to the Solanaceae, a family that furnishes many narcotic poisons. Its leaves, and the alkaloid duboisine sulphate obtained from them, are used as mydriatics, quickly paralyzing the accommodation and dilating the pupil. Its effects are less prolonged than those of atropia. Internally or by hypodermic, it produces dryness of mouth and tongue, thirst, difficulty of swallowing and loss of voice from local paralysis, frontal headache, tinnitus, vertigo, flushing of the face, dilated pupils with dim vision. Feelings of weakness, great restlessness, loss of control over the limbs, hallucinations, confusion, drowsiness, and finally delirium followed by profound comatose stupor. The article is a powerful paralyzer of the motor-sensory spinal nerves, finally reaching the heart and causing death.

Prof. O. J. Lundy, of Detroit, reported a typical case of its effects when used in the eye. Patient a robust and healthy young woman. Into each eye he put two drops solution of duboisine, 2 grains to 1 ounce, and repeated in twelve minutes, and again in an hour. In fifteen minutes from first instillation, paralysis of accommodation began, in twenty minutes it was marked and sight began to fail, in thirty-five minutes the retinal veins were enlarged, in forty-five minutes she complained of dizziness and dryness of throat. In one hour and fifteen minutes the mouth and throat were painfully dry, speech was difficult, and gait quite uncertain; and by two hours she was too dizzy to walk alone, and the burning in mouth and throat was distressing. It was not till several hours later that the poisonous effects of these minute fractions of duboisine had passed off.

ERYTHROPHLOEUM GUINENSE. Sassy Bark.

A large tree of tropical Africa. The bark furnishes a powerful poison, which is used by the natives to poison their arrow-heads, and called by them haya. It causes loss of sensibility in the nerve peripheries, loss of muscular power, local and general numbness, and intense pain, redness and swelling of adjacent parts when injected hypodermically. It follows the lines of the nerve branches inwardly from the point of injection, finally reaching the cord, developing irregular spasms, then attacking the muscles of the heart and ending in fatal systolic paralysis. Boehm, in the Archiver of Experimental Pathology, says: "After a state of paresis the animal becomes more and more restless, and there occurs an attack of extremely violent convulsions, with peculiar swimming motions, trismus, opisthotonos, spasms of the muscles of the eyes, etc. Respiration becomes slow and suffocative, and breathing ceases before the heart stops beating.

ERYTHROXYLON COCA. Coca, Cocaine.

Coca is a South American shrub, where its leaves have been used by the natives for the excitant effect they produce. The Indians there chew them much as tobacco is used, generally mingling them with some alkali, as lime or the ashes of certain plants. It is claimed that under their action the natives work or travel an day without fatigue, and this without the use of food during the day. Such claims are too extravagant for easy credence; and it is physiologically certain that an article producing such a change in the ordinary action and demands of the system, is an excitant not at all favorable to health. It is an undesirable exhilarant for civilized man. M. Mareno, in experiments on animals with coca, found that, instead of supplying the place of food, it causes a more speedy death and a greater loss of weight than starvation alone. U. S. Dispensatory. Two to three drachms of the powdered leaves is considered a dose. A tincture of 1 to 5 on diluted alcohol and a wine of 1 to 10 are used, the latter being a real tipple.

Cocaine is an alkaloidal principle found in the leaves of coca, and capable of forming soluble salts with boric, hydrochloric, lactic and nitric acids. The one commonly used is the cocaine hydrochlorate, generally spoken of simply as cocaine, and its solutions as chlorhydrate of cocaine. It is in colorless, inodorous crystals, of a slightly bitter taste, moderately soluble in cold water. A solution of 5 to 10 per cent. is the usual one for hypodermic use; and of 20 to 50 percent for local application.

Cocaine is used chiefly for its power in lessening pain, reducing the sensibility of the parts to which it is applied or injected. For this local action upon the mucous membrane of the eye it is eminent; and almost as much so about the gums in dental operations, and at other points where small surgical procedures are necessary. It acts rather promptly in blunting local sensation, and has been praised extravagantly and used enormously.

The toxic action of the article is very pronounced, and few agents are so potent for mischief, and few so uncertain as to the effects that will be produced by a given quantity. Its influence on the general nervous system is most marked, first causing excitation and then depression, beginning at the peripheries and traveling to the centers. With the insensibility it produces comes contraction of the blood-vessels; and thence local anaemia, proceeding to the brain, accompanied by muscular weakness and immobility, abolition of the reflexes, and stoppage of the heart in diastole.

Dr. J. B. Mattison, Brooklyn, gives the following list of symptoms noted in forty different cases, four of which proved fatal, the drug being applied to the eye, ear, nose, throat, gums, bowels, uterus, and under the skin: " Nausea, vomiting, headache, deafness, blindness, loss of taste and smell, profuse sweats, cold perspiration, lividity, gastric cramp; frequent, feeble, irregular, intermittent, uncountable pulse; shallow, gasping, irregular, difficult, convulsive, suspended breathing; gait, speech and swallowing greatly impaired; rigid muscles, palpitation, sense of suffocation, and great constriction about the chest; loss of motion and sensation in arms and legs, general numbness, intense restlessness, extreme prostration, giddiness, faintness, feeling of impending death; unconsciousness, convulsions; paralysis, hallucinations, mania, delusions, delirium-death. "

Similar appalling lists of symptoms have been given by many observers, and this when less than the usual safe doses were used. Injections under the skin and into the gums are peculiarly dangerous. Poisoning has been known to follow so small an amount as 77/1000 of a grain. An injection into the bladder, for vesical calculus, of a little 20 percent solution caused death almost immediately. It has come to be used habitually for the peculiar feelings of ecstacy it causes, with wild fancies and hallucinations, and it eventually brings a form of delirium tremens and actual mania. Its habitual use is liable to dethrone reason by its action on the brain substance and circulation, and few maniacs are so decidedly incurable as those brought into this condition by the cocaine habit.

EXALOINE.

Derived from acetanilid. It crystalizes in needles or tablets; scarcely soluble in cold water. It is used as an antipyretic in fevers. Its principal employment is as an analgesic in neuralgia, rheumatism and other painful affections; and an antispasmodic in chorea, etc. It is powerfully toxic, about five times as strong as antipyrine; and produces violent epileptiform convulsions, profuse salivation, rapid fall of temperature, disturbed and irregular breathing, cyanosis and prune-colored blood, and paralysis of the muscles and the heart. Average doses cause disturbance of vision, vertigo, headache, sometimes vomiting, tinnitus aurium, drowsiness, cold sweat, and disturbances of circulation; difficulty of breathing, great pallor, dilatation of the pupils, severe palpitation, and general paralysis.

FABIANA IMBRICATA. Pichi.

A member of the family Solanaceae, and tribe Nicotianae, from Chili and other parts of South America. The leaves and twigs of this shrub have been introduced into medicine: A resinous deposit abounds upon and in the leaves, which also contain a volatile oil. The article is of the terebinthinate class, with a peculiar and somewhat aromatic odor and a disagreeable pitchy taste. Like other turpentines it acts as a sharp stimulant to the kidneys, and at the same time blunts sensibility of the mucous surfaces. It has been used as a diuretic in chronic vesical catarrh, for the expulsion of cystic and renal calculi, in jaundice, and in dyspepsia, with deficient hepatic action. It may be used in decoction, an ounce in two pints, this to be taken in four equal doses in twenty-four hours. The fluid extract, not miscible with water unless an alkali is present, is given in doses of half a drachm every 6 hours. Pichi acts to the great damage of the kidneys, if continued, causing inflammation and bloody urine. On this account, like other turpentines, it is a toxic article.

GLONOIN. Trinitrine, Nitroglycerine.

This compound, usually spoken of as nitroglycerine, is prepared by adding glycerine to 1 part of nitric acid and 3 or 4 parts concentrated sulphuric acid, at a temperature made very low by artificial means. It is a bright yellow and very explosive liquid. Spiritus Glonoini, or Spirit of Nitro-Glycerine, is a one percent solution in alcohol; clear, colorless, and tasting only of alcohol, and so inclined to explosion that it must be kept in a cold place and handled very carefully.

Glonoin is used in the same places as amyl nitrite, such as angina pectoris, asthma, collapse, asphyxia, etc. Its effects are said to be somewhat more lasting than those of amyl. Its inhalation acts the same as that of amyl, and one-fourteenth of a drop has produced alarming symptoms. It causes sudden flushing of the face, headache, violent and throbbing action of the heart, and semi-unconsciousness for hours. See amyl nitrite.

GRINDELIA ROBUSTA. Gum Plant, Tar Weed.

A Compositae, chiefly from the marshes of the Pacific slope, resembling a small sunflower, exuding a gum-resin of pungently bitter taste. It is used as a stimulating anstispasmodic and expectorant in asthma, dyspnoea, whooping cough, chronic bronchitis, etc. Small doses quicken the heart and tension for a time; but soon slow the heart, decrease its strength and reduce nerve sensibility. Dr. Brubaker says: "It first lessens then destroys sensibility, the action beginning in the peripheries, then involving the trunk of the nerves, and ultimately the spinal cord. Motility is affected in the same order, paralysis beginning in the terminals. Toward the endrespir- ation becomes slower and is jerky, and death ensues by arrest of respiration. A condition of narcosis ensues as the effects of the drug develop, due to a direct impression on the cells of the cerebral lobes.

Grindelia squarrosa, ague weed, is common in the West and. South. It provokes intense neuralgic pains in the joints, eyes, brain, liver and spleen; with paralysis of respiration and great dyspnoea.

GUAIACOL.

Obtained by distilling beechwood creasote at 200 F., and treating the product with potassium and then with dilute acids. A white crystalline solid; now usually made synthetically as a darkening liquid. It has been used largely for phthisis, and is said to destroy the bacilli and promote healing of cavities. Many credible observers have failed to find it of any service. Doses ranging from 1 to 4 drops are given. Ten or more drops may came burning in the stomach, nausea and other symptoms of poisoning. Large quantities have caused rapid cyanosis, unconsciousness, vomiting, rapid pulse, anaesthesia of skin, hurried breathing, points of haemorrhage in skin; afterwards blood and albumen in urine, casts, swelling of liver and spleen, jaundice, and death on third day. Autopsy showed inflammation of stomach and bowels, haemorrhagic nephritis, degeneration of liver and heart, ecchymosis of pleurae, peritoneum, endocardium and pericardium. Such a fatal course has occured after the stomach has been relieved of the large dose by washing. It is absorbed rapidly from the stomach and skin, and by the lungs when used in inhalation.

Guaiacol carbonate is much praised as an antiseptic in typhoid, and is the essential feature of what is now known as the "Woodbridge treatment." The salt is milder than the guaiacol; but the toxic properties are yet there, and time will dampen the present high expectations.

LYSOL.

A small fraction of tar oil melts between 190° and 200°. By dissolving this in fat, and saponifying and treating with alcohol, an oily, clear and brown liquid is obtained, known as Lysol. It mixes with water, alcohol, benzine and glycerine. Its odor is somewhat like creasote. A one percent solution has a soapy feeling, and has been used as a disinfectant on the hands before operating. Mingled with sputa, pus and other discharges, its disinfecting and germicidal properties are quite marked. A five percent solution removes the odor of putrefying flesh; and it is altogether a more powerful germicide than carbolic acid, and is not irritating except in strong solutions. It is distinctly toxic; and if given internally causes subnormal fall of temperature, general depression and nephritis.

NAPHTHOL. Beta-Naphthol, Naphthalene Hydroxid.

A member in the list of coal-tar derivatives, derived from naphthalene by replacing one atom of hydrogen by an equivalent from the hydroxyl group, and hence chemically resembles the phenol or carbolic acid series. It is a crystalline powder, varying in color from white to pale yellow or huff, with a carbolic acid odor. Soluble in 1,000 parts of cold water, much more soluble in boiling water and alcohol.

It has been used largely as a disinfectant and antiseptic; in which respect it is some five or more times more potent than carbolic acid, three grains in a quart of water being sufficient to arrest the development of the so-called pathogenic germs. On this basis it has been used for intestinal disinfection in typhoid fever, 3 to 4 grains being given in capsule every two hours, with many commendations of the treatment. Also given in epidemic influenza, diarrhoea, dysentery, and low fevers with albuminous urine, it being claimed that the article will cause the albumen to disappear. Solutions have been used in conjunctivitis, otitis, chronic laryngitis, etc. It has been incorporated in soaps, 2 to 1,000, and used thus on ichthyosis, prurigo, herpes, and other skin diseases. One of the best disinfectants of its class in the sick room for faeces, urine, etc. Experiments upon animals showed it acted upon the respiratory nerves, arresting the breathing and causing death, the heart continu~ng to act some moments after respiration had ceased. It is supposed to act similarly on man, the theoretical fatal dose being 3,000 grains or more. Its toxicity is on these data feeble; but it will probably be found dangerous in much smaller doses, and is a better disinfectant than remedy.

PHENACETINE. Phenetidine, Para-acet-amido-phenetol, Para-acetphenetidine, Para-oxyethel-acetanilide.

Phenacetine is in the same coal-tar group as acetanilid. It is in colorless, tasteless, inodorous, scaly crystals; soluble in 1500 parts of cold and 80 parts of boiling water. Like its congeners, acetanilid and antipyrin; it is used as an anti neuralgic and antipyretic in rheumatism, neuralgia, hemicrania, etc. It has been prescribed lavishly and with great confidence. The toxic effects produced by it are very marked. It is productive of ptyalism, eructations, vomiting, diarrhma and toxic nephritis' and haematuria, in therapeutical doses. Prof. Frankel has seen serious effects from one-half the average dose; and an actress aged 17 died from taking one ordinary dose. Dr. Jaschke found very small doses in children caused profuse diaphoresis, intense cyanosis and symptoms of collapse. Numerous observers have found it cause excessive and alarming perspiration, extensive rashes, nausea, vertigo, chills, languor, tremors, and cyanosis. Prof. Kronig relates a case where it caused blue lip, intermittent pulse, respiratiun 32, chocolate-colored urine, cyanosis of the lips, ears, hands and feet, and yellow coloration of the body. Moderate doses given to healthy persons cause headache, dizziness, trembling of the limbs, and unsteady locomotion. Usual dose, 4 to 15 grains.

Several toxic combinations are derived from the phenetidine series, such as citropen, phenocoll, saliphen, etc.; all acting similarly to phenacetine.

PHENOCOLL.

An alkaline base obtained by acting on phenacetine with amido-acetic ether. Forms salts with acids, the hydrochloride being the phenocoll of the shops. A colorless powder dissolving in 15 parts of water. It is given as an antipyretic and antineuralgic in rheumatism, neuralgia, etc.; and applied to wounds and ulcers as an antiseptic by powder, solution, ointment, or gauze. It is readily decomposed by alkalies andcarbonates, and then acts like phenacetine. Reduces heart action, and causes death by central respiratory paralysis.

PICROTOXIN.

Colorless, odorless, shining crystals, soluble in 240 parts of cold water. It has been used for epilepsy and chorea, in doses of 1-100th of a grain, and more. A highly poisonous article, causing reduction of the heart's action, violent convulsions, stoppage of respiration and death. Its bitterness led to its use in beer, but this is prohibited by law.

PILOCARPUS PINNATIFOLIUS. Jaborandi.

Pilocarpus, a member of the rue family, is a small shrub from Brazil, with pinnate leaves a foot or more in length, the oval leaflets 3 inches long.

Its leaves have been introduced to medicine as a very active diaphoretic and sialogogue, acting quickly and with great power, pungent, and causing gastric distress. It produces enormous secretion of the salivary glands and of the sweat glands, and some increase of the lachrymal glands and the kidneys. Perspiration begins in about half an hour from an internal dose, accompanied by shivering or chilliness, pallor and pulse reduction. It has been given in acute diseases calling for perspiratory activity, as rheumatism, gout, croup and fevers; also in albuminuria, diabetes, etc. Its mode of action is by prostration of the motor nerves and voluntary muscles, weakening the heart and ending in syncope and possible paralysis. So great is the prostration during its action, that a trifling exertion may cause serious or even fatal syncope; and it is considered advisable always to have at hand some strong stimulant lest the syncope prove lethal. It leaves the system weak for some time.

At the best, the action of the agent is prostrating and dangerous. Dose of the fluid extract, 10 to 40 drops. Its active principle is alkaloidal, forming salts with muriatic and nitric acids, known as pilocarpine hydrochlorate and nitrate. Dose one-sixteenth of a grain.

PIPERAZINE. Diethylene=diamine, Dispermine.

By the action of aniline with aethylene bromide in the presence of potassium hydrate in water, there results the diphenyl-piperazine. By treating this with sulphuric acid, and distilling the product with alkalies, piperazine results. It is in lustrous, silky, white crystals or scales, very soluble in water. Outside of the body it unites readily with uric acid, forming a very soluble compound; and this fact suggested its use as a uric solvent in treating uraemia, gout and rheumatism. The reports of its employment are quite conflicting, some favoring its use and others saying it procured no worthy results. Like other phenyl combinations, it is quite likely to he decomposed in the body. In the lower animals it causes vomiting, irregular breathing and prostration, in most respects resembling the effects of carbolic acid; and reports of its. similar action on man are coming forward.

PIPER METHYSTICUM. Kava Kava, Kawa.

A member of the piperacere family, native to the Sandwich and other Pacific ocean islands. A small shrub, dicecious, with large membranous leaves and a large fibrous root or rhizome. The rhizome and base of the stalk are used, and contain an active principle called methysticin.

Kava Kava has been commended as a pungent tonic, acting largely on the mucous membranes, first increasing and then diminishing their discharges, and giving relief to suffering. It has been used in bronchial affections, catarrhs, cystitis, gonorrhoea; and some have praised it in gout, and others in erysipelas. It is used locally or inwardly, considerable doses being followed by a decided erysipelatoua eruption. The relief it gives in gonorrhcea, hronchitis, and other difficulties is of the anaesthetic character. Dose of fluid extract, 10 to 30 drops.

The toxic power of kava kava is pronounced, and it begets a form of drowsy intoxication, for which the natives of New Zealand and other isles use it, and Europeans follow their example. When first taken it produces a burning sensation and an increased flow of saliva and urine, followed by numbness that is marked and a depression of all the functions. It causes complete loss of sensibility in the mouth, throat, eye and other parts to which it may be applied; and constitutionally it produces general insensibility, diminishes and finally destroys reflex action, and causes death by paralysis. It first excites and then reduces the heart action; first stimulates and then diminishes respiration, and ends by paralyzing this function. Its principal effect is upon the spinal cord, and with this the sensory nerves. Any relief it gives is the relief of sensory paralysis.

PISCIDIA ERYTHRINA. Jamaica Dogwood.

A small tree of the family Leguminosre, native to the West Indies. For a number of years the bark of the root has engaged some professional attention, and for twelve or more years bas been of considerable prominence. It has been warmly commended in neuralgia, sick headache, rheumatism, delirium tremens, chorea, and several other forms of nervous suffering and disturbance. A safe and effectual remedy for such troubles is very desirable, and the early reports on Jamaica dogwood raised a hope that it would fill this important place. Later and more exact observations have shown it to be a peculiar and deceptive narcotic of a thoroughly dangerous character; and that the temporary relief it promotes is not of a curative nature, but is accomplished by striking down the sensorium, the heart and the respiratory apparatus. These are the three great life-centers, and piscidia gives a measure of ease at the expense of them all.

In the supplement to the Therapeutic Gazette for March, 1883, Dr. Isaac Ott reports his thorough investigations of this article, the sum of which was: In piscidia we have a drug capable of producing death by the arrest of the respiratory apparatus. It is narcotic to animals and man. It produces a tetanoid state by a stimulant action on the spinal cord; first dilates the pupils, which next contract from the asphyxia; and finally prostrates the heart. He concludes: "In the use of this drug I would like to add the caution that its surface is pleasure and its depth is death." Many other observers confirm Dr. Ott, and show Jamaica dogwood to be a peculiar and dangerous narcotic.

PYOKTANNIN. Methyl Violet.

A dye-stuff, made of a mixture of hydrochlorides of rosaniline, forming a very soluble, blue, crystalline powder. It is an active antiseptic and germicide, 2 parts in 1000 preserving paste, milk, butter, etc., almost indefinitely.

Under the germ theory of disease this property led to its use as a local application in diphtheria, epithelioma, cancer, carbuncles, foul ulcers, and similar conditions. It is quite as active in toxic as in germicidal powers, causing weak and irregular pulse, intense headache, violent and prostrating vomiting, irregular breathing, giddiness and cyanosis.

RHUS TOXICODENDRON. Poison Oak, Poison Ivy.

This species of Rhus is a shrub-like plant one to three feet high, sometimes decumbent, bearing three leaflets on a long petiole; two lateral leaflets about four inches long, broadly-ovate, pointed; terminal leaflet oval with a wedge-shaped base. Scattered from Canada to Georgia, with axillary panicles of direcious flowers; flowers small, greenish-white, June and July; fruit a round, pale-brown drupe.

Rhus radicans is a strong climbing shrub, rising to great heights upon trees, over rocks and along fences, with innumerable thread-like rootlets binding it to other objects for support. Three leaflets on long petioles; flowers small, greenish white, direcious; fruit round, pale green or whitish. Its climbing growth resembles that of the ampelopsis; but the leaflets of the latter are five instead of three; and its berries purplish-black.

Rhus venenata, swamp sumach, is a small tree 12 to 15 feet or more high; bark dark gray, on young branches and petioles red; leaves of four or five pairs ot opposite leaflets and a terminal one; leaflets oval, pointed, nearly sessile. Direcious flowers greenish, very small, in June and July; berries small, greenish-while. Frequent in swamps from Canada southward; so intensely poisonous that the wind flowing over it becomes laden with its toxic properties, which severely affect persons who come near it, though a few people handle the plant with impunity.

R. pumila is a California and Southern species about a foot high, with 9 to 13 ovate leaflets covered with a velvety pubescence beneath; fruit red, with a silky pubescence. The most poisonous of the poison sumachs. All are to be distinguished from the R. aromatica, described in the first part of this work; and they exude a juice, at first milky, but getting nearly black on exposure, which it seems impossible to remove from linen or cotton goods.

R. toxicodendron leaves have been given in palsy and cutaneous diseases. It is a harsh and irritating article, causing inflammation of the stomach and bowels with acute suffering, followed by general symptoms of narcotism. On the surface it causes intense burning, itching, redness and great swelling, resembling severe erysipelas; followed by numerous spots of vesicatiun, and finally desquamation. The suffering is severe for several days, and is best relieved by cloths wet in strong lobelia infusion and kept upon the parts. Inwardly it causes burning soreness of the throat extending to the stomach, harsh cough, thirst, high fever, nervous twitchings, deficient and irritating urine, probably a vesicular eruption, and not infrequently cerebral disturbances.

SALOL. Phenyl Salicylate.

Prepared by heating coal-tar phenol and sodium salicylate with pentachloride of phosphorus. A white crystalline powder, with a slight aromatic odor. Nearly insoluble in water; soluble in ten parts of alcohol, in ether, and fixed and volatile oils. From its great insolubility it passes through the stomach practically unchanged; but in the small intestines the alkaline condition separates it into its constituents of salicylic acid and phenol-64 per cent. of the former and 36 per cent. of the latter.

It is employed to get the antiseptic action of its two constituents in the bowels, together with the salicylic acid effect on rheumatism. It is not so effective as the salicylic acid alone; and any considerable doses will produce the poisonous effects of that acid. Its phenol makes it a highly dangerous article: and all the more if there is any renal trouble. Dose 15 grains three or more times a day. This would liberate seven-fold more carbolic acid than would be safe. Highly praised for rheum-atism, it is treacherous and dangerous.

SALOPHEN. Acetyl-par-amido-phenyl Salicylate.

Obtained by the acetification of nitro-salol; and was introduced as a substitute for salol, to avoid the serious action of the latter. In colorless, tasteless crystals, insoluble in water, soluble in alcohol and ether. It is a "new salol," used chiefly to allay the suffering of acute and chronic rheumatism, and an intestinal antiseptic in typhoid and other conditions. Some of the early reports of its effects in rheumatism were astonishing, and the agent was welcomed with enthusiasm. But experience showed that this hope had no foundation. Salophen contains about 51 per cent. of salicylic acid; and is split up by the alkaline elements of the intestines, which resolve it into salicylic acid and a phenol. The two toxic agents are thus set free, each to do its own work; the acid being the more readily absorbed, is the more marked in its effects.

If injected under the skin salophen will split up in the same manner. Its use on small animals was followed by discomfort, restlessness, haematuria, dyspnea, spasms and death. It congests the kidneys and breaks down their blood vessels. Dr. Drews says: "'While with salol the poisoning takes place exclusively from the phenol, with salophen the fatal effect-on man-is attributable to a genuine poisoning by salicylic acid." These salicylic acid effects he states as being "exhausting profuse perspiration, eruptions of sudamina, marked tinnitus, restlessness, vertigo, deafness, delirum and collapse."

SOLANUM CAROLINENSE. Horse Nettle, Bull Nettle.

A member of the Solnnacere, which includes such a large number of narcotic plants. A coarse and prickly weed, abounding on sandy soil through the Carolinas and southward, where it is often called sand-brier. In 1889 Dr. J. L. Napier wrote of it in the Medical World, relating a case of epilepsy in which a strong tincture of the fruit proved effectual. Since then it has been used in epilepsy and other convulsions. Some physicians have reported warmly in its favor, making no discrimination in their cases and not stating the underlying causes which led to the paroxysmal explosions. Others have reported entirely negative results. It acts by blunting the sensibility of the cortex; and it is said to be useless in epilepsy unless pushed to a point where it causes stupor, in which state the patient needs to be kept one, two or several days. Much was expected from it; but experience has not sustained that expectation, nor shown the relation of the article to the pathology of the disease.

STROPHANTHUS HISPIDUS.

A member of the Apocynacere, from the tropical portions of the West Coast of Africa. A woouy climber of large size, with pale-yellow flowers, producing small greyish-green or fawn-colored and hairy seeds borne in bifid and densely hirsute follicles nearly a foot long. The seeds have been introduced as a powerful cardiac stimulant, claimed to be a most effectual tonic in mitral and other valvular diseases. For such purposes it is said to be superior to digitalis. Its tincture, made with one ounce to the pint, is given in doses of 1 to 5 drops, administered cautiously because of its very great toxicity. Its active principle, strophanthin, is too dangerous for use.

As a poison, strophanthus probably has few equals in rapidity and power. It acts chiefly upon the heart as a muscle, irritating it to more forceful effort, causing systole to become very frequent and brief, with enormous increase of blood pressure and secondarily an increase of urine, and constant liability to a very sudden cessation of heart action in diastole. It causes intense burning in the esophagus and stomach, loss of appetite, and extreme gastric distress. Prof. T. R. Fraser, Edinburgh, reported, in substance, as follows, in the British Med. Jour., 1885:

Experiments prove that strophanthus causes death by paralysis of the heart. Frogs, turtles, birds, rabbits, dogs and cats are killed by it. Strophanthin produces death much more rapidly than digitaline. A solution of digitaline, one to 4000, does not stop the heart of a frog; yet of strophanthin one to 10,000,000 kills the animal.

In warm-blooded animals death occurs much sooner; and the higher in the scale of life the animal is, the more speedy is strophanthus in destroying life. In mammals, death is very rapid. In five minutes after subcutaneous injection you notice malaise, dyspnea; afterwards emesis, muscular paralysis, extreme irregularity of pulse and respiration, a violent convulsion, death. The drug acts on the heart; the heart, after death. is in a state of ventricular systole, and its muscle in a condition resembling cadaveric rigidity.

STRYCHNOS MALACCENSIS. Hoang-Nan, Tropical Bindweed.

A new species of strychnos; from Malacca and adjacent islands. Its bark has been commended as a cure for leprosy; also for constitutional syphilis, eczema and other skin diseases; and especially in recent paralysis, whether rheumatismal or syphilitic. Some of the reports are so enthusiastic as to make it seem that. failure was an impossibility. Powdered hoang-nan is given in three-grain doses three times a day; and the tincture (four parts equaling one of the bark) three to ten drops, largely diluted.

Like others of the strychnias, it is a powerful poison; and small doses soon cause muscular tremblings, tetanic spasms, and vertigo. It presently brings on a series of convulsive attacks of varying intensity, a convulsion being easily started by a touch. Between the convulsions the muscles are quivering. Dr. J. V. Shoemaker, Philadelphia, thus reports his observations on frogs, rabbits and dogs: " It soon produced severe clonic spasms, which presently assumed a tetanic character. Injected into the jugular of a dog, it caused general clonic and titanic spasms, and a rapid fall of blood pressure, beginning twenty seconds after injection. Death occurred in five minutes; the movements of respiration ceased in two minutes, three minutes before failure of the heart's action."

Others have shown that the lower extremities are first tetanized, and the highest contraction is after death. It is one of the most rapid and most uncontrollable of poisons.

SULPHONAL. Sulfonal.

Obtained by mixing acetone (from the dry distillation of calcium acetate) with anhydrous ethyl-mercaptan, and passing dry hydrochloric acid gas through the mixt.ure. The oxidized resultant yields sulphonal, which has the chemical synonym of di-ethyl-sulphon-dimethyl-methane. Permanent colorless crystals, soluble in 500 parts of cold water and 65 parts of cold alcohol; much more soluble in boiling water.

Sulphonal is praised for its efficacy in procuring sleep, relieving suffering, curing la grippe, rheumatism, headache, etc. When introduced, it was placed among the most desirable and effective hypnotics in nervous insomnia and neuralgia in general. Further observations have not sustained the encomiums given it, and the article is now little commended. Dr. J. P. Crozier has formulated the dangers of sulphonal as follows:

" It is slow in action and may be several hours in producing sleep. In a few cases the hypnotic effect has been delayed twelve and even twenty hours. It not infrequently produces delirium, followed by nausea and vomiting. Chief among the ill effects are mental excitement, nausea, vomiting, dizziness, headache, languor, exhaustion, depression, and a staggering gait. These symptoms may appear either after large or after quite small doses."

THALLINE. Thallina.

"An artificially grouped combination of coal-tar derivatives," thalline is of unusually complex constitution, prepared synthetically. It is, in its pure state, an oily fluid of a pleasant aromatic odor, forming yellowish crystals at a low temperature, of strong basic qualities. Its sulphate is the form mostly used, the tartrate being similar. These are in a yellowish-white crystalline powder, of a coumarin odor, bitter, soluble in seven parts of cold water. Thalline has been used as an antipyretic and analgesic, and for a time was pronounced a most valuable agent for reducing the temperature of all fevers. Further experience showed it to be an active poison, even while it was proclaimed, commercially, to be "a perfectly certain, safe and eligible" article. It causes vomiting, diarrhea, cyanosis and collapse; and Jaksch, who at one time favored it, says it "may be productive of dangerous and even life-imperiling symptoms." Like its congener, Kairin, it is now pretty much discarded.

THYMOL.

By submitting for a long time to a low temperature the volatile oil of some species of monarda, thyme and other plants, there crystallizes from them the article thymol. This is in large, white crystals, not unlike menthol; of a strong, thyme-like aroma, pungent taste, a caustic-like action on the lips, neutral; soluble in 1 part of alcohol, 1200 parts of water, and in fixed and volatile oils. It may be obtained in a liquid form by treating oil of thyme with solution of caustic soda, decomposing this with an acid, and distilling the thymol. It is this latter form that is mostly used, being more soluble in water.

Thymol is slightly caustic in its concentrated state, and, chemically, belongs to the carbolic acid series, but is commended by its fragrance. Largely diluted, it is used as an antiseptic in mouth washes and a wash to foul sores; but it is rarely used internally, and is likely to prove a dangerous article. Mr. Laurie, in the Lancet, reported giving one grain internally every two hours, gradually increasing to five grains, and cured two cases of chyluria dependent on filariae, for which no remedy is said to be known; but I respectfully invite attention to the agents hamamelis and sulphur, in this volume. Thymol has caused ringing in the ears, deafness, sweating, and signs of collapse; and used hypodermically in dogs, has killed them.

TRIONAL. Di-ethyl-sulphon-methyl-ethyl-methane.

This is a sulphonal analogue, an equivalent of the methyl group being substituted for one of the ethyl group. Chemically it is di-ethyl-sulphon-methyl-ethyl-methane. In flat crystals, white, shining, inodorous, bitter; soluble in 320 parts of cold water; freely soluble in hot water, hence usually given in hot tea, coffee, milk, or soup.

Trional has come into use prominently as a hypnotic, not for the relief of pain but to promote sleep in the varied forms of insomnia. In this connection it has been used in simple wakefulness, and in the sleeplessness of neurasthenia, of mental diseases, of hysterical dementia, and even of acute mania and delirium tremens. In the excitement and wakefulness incident to curing the morphine habit, it is now largely relied on by physicians who make this a specialty.

In all these relations it is said to calm the patient quickly; and to induce sleep in from half an hour to two hours, according to the severity of the case and the dose given; and this sleep is said to be calm and natural, continuing for five, seven and even ten hours. The dose ranges from 7t to 45 grains, usually given in doses of 20 to 25 grains, and this may be reduced subsequently as needed. It is said not to create a habit.

Reports are lacking as to the manner in which this article acts in procuring sleep. Looking at the general reports, as above condensed, it would seem to be a most desirable agent under very troublesome circumstances. Eminent gentlemen differ as to the form of its influence; and some have observed from it malaise, cyanosis and gastric disturbance. It generally leaves the patient very drowsy the following day. Dr. Drews, of Hamburg, noticed it causing headache, oppression in the head, weakness, nausea and ringing in the ears, continuing for several days.

USTILAGO MAIDIS. Corn Smut, Corn Ergot.

Corn smut has been used in place of ergot as a stimulant to uterine contractions in labor. In doses of 10 to 20 drops every hour or less, it is said to act effectually, without inducing the tonic rigidity and permanency of contraction that so endanger mother and child when ergot is given. It has also been commended in uterine hemorrhages, amenorrhoea, and other troubles incident to reduced uterine tonicity. Dr. J. Mitchell, University of Pennsylvania, made a thorough study of the drug, and reported his observations in the Therapeutic Gazette of 1886, p. 223; from which the following points are condensed:

The most characteristic effect of the drug is one of paralysis. It diminishes and finally abolishes all reflex action. This is mainly on the sensory portion of the spinal cord, first; and the motor nerves, though for a time unaffected, are ultimately depressed and finally paralyzed. Before these effects are fully developed, convulsions commonly occur, which seem to be of spinal rather than of muscular origin. The ultimate action of the ustilago maidis upon the nervous system is that of a universal depressant, producing diminution and final extinction of all reflex and volitional phenomena, with the early induction of narcotism. The loss of reflex activity is due to the paralysis of the sensory portion of the cord.

The motor portion of the cord is also depressed, as well as the motor nerves. It is also probable that the sensory nerves share in the general paralysis. Death is due to arrest of respiration, though in exceptional cases it may be due to the diastolic arrest of the heart. "

CONTENTS.

3690726R00044

Printed in Great Britain
by Amazon.co.uk, Ltd.,
Marston Gate.